# Caring for Children and Families

D1300407

# Caring for Children and Families

*Edited by*
**I. PEATE**
**L. WHITING**

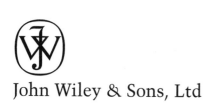

John Wiley & Sons, Ltd

### Other Wiley Editorial Offices

John Wiley & Sons Inc., 111 River Street, Hoboken, NJ 07030, USA

Jossey-Bass, 989 Market Street, San Francisco, CA 94103-1741, USA

Wiley-VCH Verlag GmbH, Boschstr. 12, D-69469 Weinheim, Germany

John Wiley & Sons Australia Ltd, 42 McDougall Street, Milton, Queensland 4064, Australia

John Wiley & Sons (Asia) Pte Ltd, 2 Clementi Loop #02-01, Jin Xing Distripark, Singapore
129809

John Wiley & Sons Canada Ltd, 6045 Freemont Blvd, Mississauga, ONT, L5R 4J3

Wiley also publishes its books in a variety of electronic formats. Some content that appears in
print may not be available in electronic books.

### Library of Congress Cataloging-in-Publication Data

Caring for children and families / edited by Ian Peate, Lisa Whiting.
    p.   ;   cm.
    Includes bibliographical references and index.
    ISBN-13: 978-0-470-01970-2 (pbk. : alk. paper)
    ISBN-10: 0-470-01970-0 (pbk. : alk. paper)
    1. Pediatric nursing.  I. Peate, Ian.  II. Whiting, Lisa. [DNLM:  1. Pediatric
Nursing – methods.  2. Family.
WY 159 C2767 2006]
RJ245.C37 2006
618.92′00231 – dc22

                                                                          2006004385

### A catalogue record for this book is available from the British Library

ISBN-13  978-0-470-01970-2
ISBN-10  0-470-01970-0

Typeset by SNP Best-set Typesetter Ltd., Hong Kong
Printed and bound in Great Britain by TJ International Ltd, Padstow, Cornwall

This book is printed on acid-free paper responsibly manufactured from sustainable forestry in
which at least two trees are planted for each one used for paper production.

For all the children and families for whom we have the privilege of caring

# Contents

# About the Editors

**Ian Peate EN(G) RGN DipN (Lond) RNT BEd(Hons) MA(Lond) LLM**
**Address for correspondence:**
Associate Head of School
School of Nursing and Midwifery
Faculty of Health and Human Sciences
University of Hertfordshire
Hatfield
Hertfordshire AL10 9AB
Ian began his nursing career in 1981 at Central Middlesex Hospital, becoming an Enrolled Nurse working in an intensive care unit. He later undertook three years' student nurse training at Central Middlesex and Northwick Park Hospitals, becoming a Staff Nurse then a Charge Nurse. He has worked in nurse education since 1989. His key areas of interest are nursing practice and theory, sexual health and HIV/AIDS. He is currently Associate Head of School. His portfolio centres on recruitment and marketing and professional academic development within the School of Nursing and Midwifery.

**Lisa Whiting MSc BA (Hons) RGN RSCN RNT LTCL**
**Address for correspondence:**
Senior Lecturer, Children's Nursing
School of Nursing and Midwifery
Faculty of Health and Human Sciences
University of Hertfordshire
Hatfield
Hertfordshire AL10 9AB
Lisa completed the four-year RGN/RSCN programme at the Queen Elizabeth Medical Centre, Birmingham in 1983. She gained a range of paediatric clinical experience, developing her career within the area of critical care nursing and becoming a Ward Sister on the children's cardiac intensive care unit at Guy's Hospital. Lisa has worked in education for a number of years, teaching students undertaking a variety of children's nursing programmes. In addition, she has studied academically and nurtured an interest in child health promotion.

# About the Contributors

**Cathy Cairns RGN RSCN BSc(Hons) PGCert**
Deputy Director of Nursing and Practice Governance
**Address for correspondence:**
Hertfordshire Partnership NHS Trust
Trust Head office
99 Waverly Road
St Albans
Hertfordshire AL3 5TL
Cathy has held various clinical, educational and management roles within children's services in Nottingham, London and Bristol. Cathy's professional interests are diverse and encompass anything which contributes to the provision of safe and effective care.

**Mary Donnelly SRN RSCN DipHEd PGCertEd BSc(Hons)**
**Address for correspondence:**
Senior Lecturer in Children's Health
School of Nursing and Midwifery
Faculty of Health and Human Sciences
University of Hertfordshire
Hatfield
Hertfordshire AL10 9AB
Mary began her nursing career in 1978 training to be a state-registered nurse at Edgware General Hospital's School of Nursing. On completion of training she became a Staff Nurse in the accident and emergency department at Edgware General and later became a Senior Staff Nurse in the same hospital's children's ward. In 1986 she became an industrial nursing officer, but returned to accident and emergency nursing in 1990. While working in the accident and emergency department in Barnet General Hospital, Mary studied for her second registration as a Registered Sick Children's Nurse becoming an Accident and Emergency Sister and Paediatric Nurse specialist for the same hospital. In 2001 she became a Nurse Facilitator for the North Central London Workforce Development Confederation and later went on to become the acting lead nurse for the cadet nursing scheme for the same organisation. She has been employed as a Lecturer in children's health at the University of Hertfordshire since 2003.

**Liz Gormley-Fleming RGN RSCN BSc(Hons) PGCert MA**
**Address for Correspondence:**
University of Hertfordshire
College Lane
Hatfield
Hertfordshire AL10 9AB
Liz trained and worked in Dublin as an RSCN before arriving in the UK in 1990 to work at Northwick Park Hospital, initially as an RGN but then moved to Children's Services where she undertook many roles, from Staff Nurse to Lead Nurse, finally leaving the Trust in 2001. Liz also worked in Northern Ireland for a brief time during the nineties. Her interest in nurse education led her to her next role as Clinical Facilitator in Hertfordshire Partnership NHS Trust before finally moving into higher education full time. Her areas of interests are clinical-skills development, the legal and ethical aspects of child health nursing and evidence-based care.

**Dee Harris RGN RSCN DPNS SNP BSc(Hons)(HV) MA(Herts) PGDipHE ENB 998 ENB 934 ENB 415**
**Address for correspondence:**
Senior Lecturer
School of Nursing and Midwifery
Faculty of Health and Human Sciences
University of Hertfordshire
Hatfield
Hertfordshire AL10 9AB
Dee began her nursing career in 1979 at Queen Elizabeth II Hospital, Welwyn Garden City. Following this adult introduction, Dee followed a post-registration pathway at Great Ormond Street Hospital and has worked with children ever since in both acute and community settings. Her experience also includes paediatric intensive care and health visiting; a number of her posts were in a senior capacity and included a child-protection role at named-nurse level. Dee has worked in nurse education since 2002; her key areas of interest include legal, professional and ethical issues in child care, children's rights and care delivery and management, which include the virtual teaching of skills. Her portfolio centres on pre- and post-registration learning, including safeguarding children and interprofessional facilitation in child protection.

**Patricia Harwood RGN RSCN DipN(Education) RNT AdvancedDip in Curriculum and Teaching BA BSc(Hons) MSc**
**Address for correspondence:**
Senior Lecturer
School of Nursing and Midwifery

Faculty of Health and Human Sciences
University of Hertfordshire
Hatfield
Hertfordshire AL10 9AB

Patricia gained her RGN qualification in May 1971 and registered with the Medical Dental and Allied Professions Council of Rhodesia (now Zimbabwe). She worked as a Staff nurse gaining experience in medical and surgical nursing. In August 1973 she qualified as a midwife and registered with the Medical Council. Patricia worked for a short while as a midwife but became increasingly interested in infant and child care, and transferred to a general paediatric ward as a Staff Nurse and later as a Sister. In 1983 in the UK she worked as a nurse teacher at the Mid-Hertfordshire School of Nursing, and later as a Senior Lecturer with the University of Hertfordshire. Patricia graduated with her RSCN from Great Ormond Street Hospital in 1993. Her special interests are child studies and simulation, biosciences in nursing and nursing practice.

**Lyn Karstadt MA BA RGN RSCN RNT DipN(Lond) CertEd(FE)**
**Address for correspondence:**
Head of School & Associate Dean of Faculty
School of Nursing and Midwifery
Faculty of Health and Human Sciences
University of Hertfordshire
Hatfield
Hertfordshire AL10 9AB

Lyn completed her RGN in Nottingham and her RSCN at Great Ormond Street Hospital. She spent time working at Great Ormond Street in a range of Staff Nurse positions before moving to Mount Vernon Hospital in Middlesex as a Ward Sister on a general children's ward. Lyn moved into nurse education in 1983 and has experience teaching students undertaking a variety of nursing programmes in several educational institutions. Her academic interest is in nurse education, particularly curriculum structures. Lyn has been Head of the School of Nursing and Midwifery at the University of Hertfordshire since 2002.

**Billie Kell BSc(Hons) RN(Child) PGCE PGDip RHV**
**Address for correspondence:**
School of Nursing and Midwifery
Faculty of Health and Human Sciences
University of Hertfordshire
Hatfield
Hertfordshire AL10 9AB

Billie began her nursing career in 1997 having undertaken a degree programme in nursing at De Montfort University in Leicester. She commenced working at the Leicester Royal Infirmary's Children's Hospital on both the Emergency Medical Assessment Unit and a surgical ward. She then worked as a School Nurse in the community setting. In 1999 she returned to the Leicester Royal Infirmary to work for the Critical Care and Theatres Directorate as Senior Paediatric Day Care Practitioner, until moving into nurse education at the University of Wales College of Medicine. In 2002 she qualified as a Health Visitor and worked in this capacity until April 2004, when she returned to the field of nurse education. Her key areas of interest are child health, in particular health promotion and effective collaboration working. She is currently a Senior Lecturer at the School of Nursing and Midwifery.

**Sue Miller MSc BSc(Hons) RGN RSCN DN CertEd**
**Address for correspondence:**
Senior Lecturer, Children's Nursing
School of Nursing and Midwifery
Faculty of Health and Human Sciences
University of Hertfordshire
Hatfield
Hertfordshire AL10 9AB
Sue completed her initial nurse education programme at Northwick Park Hospital and later undertook the RSCN course at Great Ormond Street Hospital. She gained a range of clinical experience, developing her career within the area of general and community children's nursing. Sue has worked in nurse education for a number of years, teaching both pre- and post-registration students undertaking a variety of children's nursing programmes. In addition, she has studied academically and has a particular interest in child health promotion, caring for children with special needs and those with long-term health problems.

**Julie Robinson**
Senior Hospital Play Specialist
**Address for correspondence:**
Coxen Ward
Royal National Orthopaedic Hospital
Brockley Hill
Stanmore
Middlesex HA7 4LP
Relevant qualifications: Child Psychology, Sociology, PPA Leader's certificate, Makaton signing certificates levels 1 & 2, Distinction in Hospital Play Specialism

## Helen Russell-Johnson RN RSCN RNT BSc(Hons) MA

Senior Lecturer Children's Nursing and Interprofessional Learning Coordinator
School of Nursing and Midwifery
Faculty of Health and Human Sciences
University of Hertfordshire
Hatfield
Hertfordshire AL10 9AB
Helen started her nursing career in 1971 at the Royal Salop Infirmary in Shrewsbury and then moved to London in 1976 to undertake her Registered Sick Children's Nurse and Diploma in Nursing at Great Ormond Street Hospital. After working there as both a Staff Nurse and a Sister, she moved into education at the Charles West School of Nursing, first as a Clinical Teacher then as a Tutor. Following a break to raise a family, she returned to nursing and teaching in 1991. Her main areas of interest are child law, child protection, adolescent care and child and adolescent mental health.

## Peter Vickers CertEd DipCD SRN RSCN BA PhD

**Address for correspondence:**
Senior Lecturer – Child Nursing
School of Nursing and Midwifery
Faculty of Health and Human Sciences
University of Hertfordshire
Hatfield
Hertfordshire AL10 9AB
Peter began teaching in both primary and secondary education in 1961 and was a student at St Luke's Teacher Training College, Exeter, and later undertook an advanced course at the Cardiff College of Art, University of Wales. Initially specialising in the education of children with special needs, and becoming the Deputy Head of a school for children with severe behavioural problems, he then specialised in the teaching of arts and crafts. Following four years' working with the Army, he commenced nurse training at the York School of Nursing, undertaking further studies at the Charles West School of Nursing, Great Ormond Street. He worked as a Staff Nurse, Charge Nurse and later Clinical Nurse Specialist for Paediatric Immunology. Following this, he worked as Clinical Nurse Manager for Paediatrics at Newcastle General Hospital, commencing his PhD studies, before entering nurse education in 1992. Subsequently, he again worked in the clinical area, in the Paediatric Unit at the Luton & Dunstable Hospital, before commencing his present position at the University of Hertfordshire. Peter was awarded his doctorate in 1999 for his research into children who had survived bone marrow transplants for immune deficiency disorders, and their families, in the UK and Germany. He now teaches the biosciences, immunology and immunodeficiency, children's health, and research, as well as undertaking his own research studies.

# Acknowledgements

We would like to thank all of our colleagues for their help, support, comments and suggestions. We thank Anthony Peate, who produced the illustrations.

Lisa would particularly like to thank her children, husband and parents for their continued support, encouragement and love.

Ian would like to thank his partner for all of his continued support and encouragement.

# 1 Introduction

## I. PEATE AND L. WHITING

This text has been written as a resource for those who provide health care for children and their families. Contributors to the book are experts from a range of backgrounds – both in practice and academia. The contributors firmly believe, that the child comes first and foremost; they believe that each child is a unique person with individual needs and aspirations – this stance is clearly reflected in each chapter of the book.

Children deserve the best possible care, and this cannot be provided unless there is an understanding of the context of children's lives, both in the community at large and within healthcare settings. The concept of partnership focuses upon the need to deliver paediatric care in collaboration with the child and the family. This text encourages the reader to apply this approach to care delivery in any situation in which they may be working. Chapter 2 emphasises the importance of this, looking beyond a disease-orientated approach to one where the child and her or his family are a clear and central unit.

The principal audience of this text are nursing students, and especially those who are undertaking NVQ/SNVQ, Access to Nursing and Cadet nursing programmes of study. It is not, however, a comprehensive book about children's nursing, and, as a result, the reader is encouraged to identify further topics of importance that have not been considered here. Within the text the terms 'nurse', 'student' and 'nursing' have been adopted. The terms and the philosophies applied to this book can be adapted to suit a number of healthcare workers at various levels and in a range of settings in order to develop caring skills.

The book presents up-to-date information that the aspiring nurse or child healthcare provider requires in order to begin to understand how to help children and families, in both the institutional setting (for example the hospital) and the community (for example the child's own home). The material is organised in such a way that it reflects contemporary practice in a user-friendly manner; in addition, information is related to clinical practice issues that may be experienced when working with children and their families. It is not envisaged that the text be read from cover to cover in one sitting; it has been designed to be used as a reference book (a resource, a reader) either in the clinical setting, classroom or in your own home.

*Caring for Children and Families*. Edited by I. Peate and L. Whiting
© 2006 John Wiley & Sons Ltd

The text should be seen as a handbook or a manual that has a sound evidence base, and one that will challenge and encourage the reader to develop a questioning approach to care provision. It emphasises the integration of theory and practice. To get the most out of this book you are strongly encouraged to attend all of your classes associated with your current programme of study, using this text to supplement and support your theoretical and clinical learning.

Much of the discussion is placed against the backdrop of the Children Act 2004 and the National Service Framework for Children, Young People and Maternity Services (DH and DfES, 2004). Other key documents, publications and statutes are also used to inform debates.

The overarching aims are to help the reader to understand the fundamental aspects of care in order to facilitate safe and effective practice – to stimulate thought and to generate discussion. This will encourage the development of paediatric caring skills underpinned with a sound knowledge base. This is a foundation text that will enable personal growth in relation to child health care.

## TERMS USED

Often a difficult task when writing a textbook is the choice of the terms to be used. 'Patient' is the expression that is commonly used within the NHS and on occasions has been adopted in this text. It is acknowledged that not everyone supports the use of the passive concept associated with this term, but it is used here in the knowledge that it is widely understood; it may apply to the family as well as the child. There are other expressions that might have been chosen, for example 'service user', 'client' or 'consumer'; however, where appropriate, 'child' and 'family' have been the terms of choice.

The phrase 'carer' has been utilised within the book. This term is used to describe those who look after children, whether they be ill, healthy or have a disability. 'Carer' has many interpretations and may refer to an employed healthcare provider or someone who provides care that is unpaid. It has been estimated that there are approximately six million unpaid carers in the UK (Carers UK, 2005); this figure includes parents, grandparents and siblings who are looking after sick children.

## THE ACTIVITIES

Each chapter has 'activities' included, which have been integrated to help, encourage and motivate you to determine your learning and progress. Some of the activities presented will provide you with possible responses to the questions set. Others do not; they are there to support your learning, to persuade you to delve deeper and further your understanding of the topic. Chapter 6 provides a different approach and includes 'review questions' to urge you to check your learning as you go along. The questions that have been set in Chapter 6 are followed by model answers.

## THE CHAPTERS

This text does not attempt to address every aspect of child health care. The chapters have been arranged in an attempt to provide insight into the complexities of providing care to children and their families. This book aims to provide you with a fundamental understanding of some of the issues that may impinge on a child's well-being.

Chapter 2 sets the scene and emphasises the importance of fostering good working relationships with children and their families. The value of key concepts, such as 'partnership', is considered and debated in detail. The diversity of the family is addressed, together with the necessity of embracing a range of family members in the child's care (for example siblings and grandparents).

Failure to communicate with children and their families has been seen as a major obstacle to effective care. In Chapter 3 the focus will be centred on effective communication strategies that may be used when caring for the child and family (for example processes and forms of communication). The chapter explores how children communicate with others, stressing that mutual respect and trust are key components (Sokal-Gutierrez and Dooling, 2005).

The healthcare worker never operates in isolation; he or she is a part of a multidisciplinary team and effective communication within this team is vital if the child and the child's family are to receive the best quality care. Chapter 4 builds upon the discussion in Chapter 3. Caring for well or sick children is challenging and the student needs to liaise with a range of health- and social-care professionals from various statutory and voluntary agencies. Those health- and social-care professionals and their roles are described.

Caring for the child and the family will involve health-promotion activities. Chapter 5 addresses health promotion using a child-centred approach. Fulfilling a child's health potential is central to care, and this chapter discusses health-promotion strategies, considering some of the special health needs of children and how families may be empowered.

A wide range of issues related to child health and illness are addressed in this text, and Chapter 6 describes childhood anatomy and physiology, identifying how this may predispose to disease, for example fundamental anatomy and physiology of the child's respiratory tract is outlined. This is followed by a discussion of potential difficulties that the child may encounter as a result of their immaturity – key examples include asthma and bronchiolitis.

Expanding upon the issues already raised, Chapter 7 contextualises the information provided. The reader is made aware that the accurate assessment of the child, correct interpretation of data and the provision of safe and effective care are essential skills that the student should strive to achieve. Ideally, both Chapters 6 and 7 should be read in sequence to inform understanding of the complexities associated with monitoring and assessing the needs of the child.

Chapter 8 uses a developmental approach to address the importance of play. An outline of 'normal' child development is provided, while the socio-economic issues associated with, and impinging upon, play are described. The impact that illness has on a child and the ability to actively engage in play is explored.

Maintaining safety is a fundamental aspect of child health care, and Chapter 9 highlights some of the main issues. There are three significant components of this chapter: the supervised administration of medicines, the safe moving, handling and positioning of children, and effective infection-control practices. These are areas of practice that are encountered on a daily basis. It is therefore imperative that health carer providers have a good level of underpinning knowledge – this chapter will facilitate this.

Following on from maintaining safety, Chapter 10 considers accident prevention. Accidents are the primary cause of death among children aged between 1 and 5 years (DH, 2002a, 2002b). A detailed discussion that is related to child development provides information that may help to reduce the number of accidents that occur to children in both the community and hospital setting.

Child-protection issues, described in Chapter 11, make clear that safeguarding children is an essential aspect of all child health care practice – 'The Child First and Always'. Policies and procedures that are in place to protect the child and identify the child 'at risk' are highlighted. Examples are used to explain, and provide insight into, this complex and sensitive aspect of care provision.

Issues associated with the law, ethics and morals are discussed in Chapter 12. Insight into some key statutory legislation that governs child care is provided; in addition, there is focus upon the legal ramifications in such a way that the reader is able to relate and apply them to practice. Once again, scenarios are utilised to illustrate points and to give added clarity.

Finally, Chapter 13 adopts a career-advice approach to encourage the reader to take the next steps to develop her or his skills and to consider professional registration as a nurse. A range of professional issues are detailed, including the role and responsibility of the Nursing and Midwifery Council, the Code of Professional Conduct, the important concept of confidentiality and professional regulation.

A glossary of terms and abbreviations is provided to further facilitate personal learning and understanding.

The contributors have enjoyed the challenge that this book has provided. We hope that you find the chapters stimulating and thought-provoking, but, most importantly, we hope that children and families in your care will benefit as a result of your learning.

## REFERENCES

Carers UK (2005) *A Manifesto for Carers*. London: Carers UK.

Department of Health (DH) (2002a) *Accidents are not Inevitable: Government sets priorities for action.* London: DH.

Department of Health (DH) (2002b) *Preventing Accidental Injury: Priorities for action.* London: DH.

Department of Health and Department for Education and Skills (DH/DfES) (2004) *National Service Framework for Children, Young People and Maternity Services.* London: DH/DfES.

Sokal-Gutierrez K and Dooling M (2005) The health care professional as a consultant to child care programs. In: American Academy of Pediatrics (eds) *Health in Child Care: A manual for health professionals*. Elk Grove Village: American Academy of Pediatrics. Chapter 14, pp. 219–234.

# 2 Children and their Families

**L. WHITING**

## INTRODUCTION

There is no doubt that children are frequent users of healthcare provision. The Department of Health (DH) (2002) suggests that the majority of sick children encounter common problems (such as respiratory illness, fever, diarrhoea and vomiting and minor injuries); however, others have a range of complex physical and emotional needs. The care and management of sick children may be met in a variety of environments including hospitals, home and school – it is essential that the different aspects of a child's life are considered when care is provided to ensure that they feel comfortable and that continuity of care is provided.

This chapter provides an introduction to working with children and their families, exploring a range of issues that are fundamental to care. Where the term 'child' is used, it will refer to individuals below the age of 19 years, including babies, children and young people (DH and DfES, 2004). Although it is recognised that these groups have differing needs, this chapter discusses core aspects of practice that are pertinent to all ages. First of all, the concept of the 'family', the central element of most children's lives, will be explored; consideration will then be given to some of the challenges and concerns that face families and how knowledge of these issues may enable the healthcare professional to enhance care provision. In addition, key historical information will be given to facilitate the understanding of the development of practice and the current healthcare service.

## THE 'FAMILY'

On their fiftieth anniversary, the United Nations in its Universal Declaration of Human Rights (1998) reiterated that the family is:

> the natural and fundamental group unit of society and is entitled to protection by society and the state. [Article 16(3)]

*Caring for Children and Families.* Edited by I. Peate and L. Whiting
© 2006 John Wiley & Sons Ltd

Most children are born into a family (Rutherford, 1998). As this normally provides the stability and security that is the lynchpin to their development, a thorough understanding of family function and structure is imperative. However, the nature of the family can vary considerably, and as a result it is difficult to offer a precise clarification of the term.

Murdoch, an eminent sociologist, offers a definition that is frequently quoted:

> A social group characterised by common residence, economic co-operation and reproduction. It includes adults of both sexes, at least two of whom maintain a socially approved sexual relationship and one or more children, own or adopted, of the sexually cohabiting adults. (Murdoch, 1949, cited by Taylor et al., 1995, p. 233)

It could be argued that this view reflected society at the time of writing but does not reflect the diversity of lifestyles that are now prevalent in the twenty-first century. Richards (1995) offers a more contemporary stance by suggesting that families are likely to consist of people who are interconnected, have emotional bonds and psychologically meaningful social interactions. This perspective would certainly embrace the wide range of family systems in which children are reared in the UK. Jacqueline Wilson, a widely read children's author, has reflected this in her books by writing stories that embrace alternative family structures. Although her work is fiction, her focus is upon the child's perspective, reading her books can provide valuable introductory insight for adults. Whatever the organisation of the family, most people still consider it to be the most important element in their lives (Bernardes, 1997). This view is reiterated by the European Parliament, Council of the European Union and European Commission (2000) in the Charter of Fundamental Rights, which states that everyone has the right to have their family life respected (Article 7) and that the 'right to found a family shall be guaranteed' (Article 9, p. 10).

Rutherford (1998) suggests that there is wide acknowledgement by both lay people and psychologists that the family has a significant impact upon children in relation to their growth, development and nurturing. As a result, the family will have tremendous insight into the uniqueness of the child and their individual needs – it is therefore essential that the care of the sick child is considered within the context of the family (this will be further discussed later in the chapter). The majority of children are reared within a family unit, and this influences their development, maturation and understanding of the world at large. Within the family, the child normally feels secure, familiar, comfortable and loved; therefore working with children necessitates working with their families and understanding their needs (Chapter 11 will discuss child-protection issues relating to the family).

There would appear to be wide consensus that the family is fundamental to the formation of society; however, family structure and diversity have changed considerably during the last century and many of the children receiving health care today do not live within a traditional family unit.

---

**Activity**
*Spend a little time thinking of factors that have influenced family structure and dynamics in the twenty-first century.*

---

You may have identified some of the following.

- There is an increasing elderly population; therefore children may form close relationships with their grandparents, great-grandparents and even great-great-grandparents. In addition, this could lead to further family stress if these ageing relatives have health problems of their own.
- The child-bearing age has widened over recent years. Teenage pregnancy has increased, with UNICEF (2001) stating that the UK has the highest rate in Western Europe. Many of these mothers have not formed a 'couple identity' with the child's father. At the same time, there are growing numbers of more mature parents – the approach and insight into child rearing will therefore vary enormously.
- Parents are now able to use alternative methods of conception, such as surrogacy, *in vitro* fertilisation and sperm donation. As a result, it is no longer unusual for a child to have two parents of the same gender.
- The UK is a multicultural and multiracial society. As a result, there is a vast array of differing family structures.
- Marriage is now no longer viewed by everyone as a necessity for the upbringing of children. In addition, adults may have a number of partners throughout their lives; therefore children may be reared by people who are not their genetic parents.
- Many parents work; therefore children may form close relationships with others, including the childminder, friends and their pets – the child may perceive these to be important family members.

It can be seen from the above points that within the twenty-first century in the UK, families are complex structures which have developed a variety of new forms (Carling, 2002). It is therefore imperative that the care which is offered to children and their families is holistic and individualised.

---

**Activity**
*It is important to recognise that healthcare professionals are also from a range of family structures. Think about your own family background and consider how this may influence the care that you provide.*

---

You may have highlighted factors such as:

- culture
- race
- ethnicity

- constituency of family members
- roles of family members
- family environment.

Recognising personal attributes is essential; it is only once this has been done that the healthcare professional can learn to respect others and to provide care in a non-judgemental and non-discriminatory manner.

## THE REACTION OF THE FAMILY TO THEIR SICK CHILD

Understanding how families may respond to a child's illness enables the healthcare professional to appreciate potential psychological and physical needs and to plan care appropriately. Families may react to their child's illness in a variety of ways; some of the most common responses are identified in Table 2.1.

---

**Activity**
*Parental reactions to a child's illness will vary tremendously, but there are a number of factors that may influence their response. Take a moment to think of issues that could have an effect.*

---

You may have considered:

- the seriousness of the child's illness;
- previous experiences of illness (either their own or their child's);
- medical procedures involved in the diagnosis and treatment of the child;
- support networks that are available (e.g. friends, family, other parents);
- personal coping abilities;
- additional stresses on the family system;
- cultural and religious beliefs;
- communication patterns among family members.

Clearly, when working with children, it is important to understand why and how families may react to a child's illness if appropriate care is to be provided. Building a therapeutic relationship and providing the opportunity to listen to both children and parents will help to develop insight into individual needs.

## PARENTING IN PUBLIC

It is essential to recognise that a child's illness may provoke extremely high levels of anxiety within the whole family. While it is acknowledged that parents have expert knowledge about their children and are capable of providing 'expert' care (Lowton, 2002), they may still feel that they are being watched by healthcare professionals and that their actions are being judged. Since this

**Table 2.1** Possible reactions of the family to their sick child

**Parental reactions**
- **Disbelief:** this is particularly common when the illness has a sudden onset, if the condition has a potential to be life threatening or if it is a long-term chronic problem.
- **Guilt:** Some parents will blame themselves for the child's illness. This may be expected when the child has suffered an accident, such as a scald – the parent may feel that they weren't vigilant enough. However, parents do also sometimes wonder if their child is sick because of an inherited genetic predisposition or because of lifestyle influences that they may have had some control over (for example poor diet or lack of exercise).
- **Anger:** This emotion may be exacerbated if treatment or care does not appear to be progressing as expected. Healthcare professionals are the people who are immediately available and who may feel the brunt of this anger – it is important to keep this in perspective and not to feel that the attack is personal.
- **Fear:** Many parents have had little previous experience of health care – perhaps the last time was the joyful event of the birth of their child. As a result, they may feel lonely, insecure and frightened. Working with the parent and providing as much information as possible will help.
- **Frustration:** Parents may, for example, become extremely frustrated if they have to wait several hours to see a doctor. Possible feelings of exhaustion and helplessness in relation to their expected role will not help. Once again, spending time with the parent and explaining the plan of care will assist.
- **Depression:** Parents may feel that they are unable to cope with their sick child as well as other family commitments. Hospital stay for children has been considerably reduced in recent years, and many children are now cared for within the community setting; so healthcare professionals may not always be immediately aware of the parent's distress. The nurturing of a therapeutic relationship is imperative so that appropriate support (and possible referral to other agencies) can be offered.

**Sibling reactions**
Sibling reactions to a sister's or brother's illness may include anger, resentment, jealousy and guilt. Various factors may influence the effects of the child's illness on siblings:

- **Fear:** This may be because they think that they may also become ill, but they may also fear losing their parent(s) if more time is being spent with a sibling.
- **Age:** A young child may have particular difficulty in understanding the child's illness.
- **Close relationship to sick sibling:** It is important to acknowledge that, while siblings may quarrel, close bonds frequently exist and these should not be underestimated.
- **Out-of-home residence:** The sibling may need to stay with another family member or friend if their sibling is hospitalised; this could provoke a range of reactions if they don't fully appreciate the reason for this.
- **Minimum explanation of the sick child's illness:** If siblings are not kept informed about the sick child, they may draw incorrect conclusions – this can lead to nightmares and disruptive behaviour if, for example, they believe that the child's condition is more serious than it actually is.
- **Perceived changes in parenting:** Parents may be preoccupied with their child's illness, causing alteration in their mood – siblings may think that they are to blame for this.

**Table 2.2** Areas of concern identified by parents of hospitalised children *(adapted from Teare and Smith, 2004)*

- listening to parents
- the stress of staying with a child in hospital
- feeling safe
- waiting
- parents as partners in care

is probably not the case, it is important that the family is provided with the necessary guidance, support and education to enable them to participate in the care of their sick child in a confident and competent manner.

Teare and Smith (2004) conducted focus-group discussions with parents of hospitalised children as part of a research study in Bradford. The aim was to highlight good practice and to improve aspects of service delivery that were of concern to the parents. Their findings indicated that parents identified five key areas (Table 2.2); these will now be discussed in more depth.

## LISTENING TO PARENTS

Teare and Smith (2004) identify the importance of communicating with the child and family. The majority of parents who have a sick child have not previously encountered their current situation. As a result, they will be anxious and uncertain of their role and the expectations that healthcare professionals have of them. It is clearly vital to listen to parents so that concerns can be identified and therapeutic relationships developed.

---

**Activity**
*Think of a situation when someone made assumptions about your needs without listening to your requirements.*

---

Perhaps you felt a loss of control or inadequate, angry, frustrated, tearful or sad. None of these are positive emotions, and this can subsequently influence self-esteem, confidence levels and your ability to carry out tasks effectively. Parents of sick children may experience similar emotions if they are not listened to.

Carter (2004, p. 179) reminds us that 'the best teachers, providing that we take notice of them, are the children and parents'; the listening role acknowledges the parents' expert knowledge about their child and that they have far more insight into the child's usual behaviour than the healthcare professional – using this knowledge will further enhance care. Making time to talk to the whole family is essential; some family members, such as fathers who may be at work during the day, can feel neglected. Likewise, siblings may feel that the sick child is receiving more attention than they are and they may not fully appreciate the underlying rationale for this; listening to them may help you to understand their perspective. (This aspect of care is discussed further in Chapter 3.)

## THE STRESS OF STAYING WITH A HOSPITALISED CHILD

The opportunity for parents (in particular, mothers) to be resident with their hospitalised child is not a new concept. Although relatively few children were admitted to hospital in the nineteenth century, it was not unusual for them to be accompanied by their mother, who would remain with them until discharge home (Lindsay, 2003). This certainly enabled the child to receive the care that they required, there was little opposition to the idea and it appears to have been routine practice. Parents who were not able to stay with their child were actively encouraged to visit as much as possible as this was felt to be important for the child's well-being and also provided the opportunity to teach parenting skills (*The Times*, 1874, cited by Lindsay, 2003). It was not until towards the end of the nineteenth century that hospitals began to slowly exclude parents from the ward areas. There were two main reasons for this change in attitude; first of all, psychologists of the time felt that children became too distressed by their families visiting and, secondly, there was concern that infection would spread far more rapidly. By the 1930s the majority of hospitals across the UK were not allowing parental access unless the child had a prolonged (usually more than four-week) admission.

In the 1940s there was a gradual movement towards welcoming parents back to hospital wards. In the late 1940s and throughout the 1950s two people played a key role in this change – John Bowlby (an eminent psychiatrist who specialised in child psychology) and James Robertson (a social worker). In 1953 Robertson made a film entitled *A 2-year-old goes to hospital* (Robertson, 1958) that highlighted the effects of hospitalisation on young children (2 to 5 years of age) if a parent was not present. The stages that Robertson identified are highlighted in Table 2.3 – you may occasionally see these if a child does not have a familiar person with them. In addition, a group of mothers founded an organisation called the National Association for the Welfare of Children in Hospital (NAWCH); this still exists but has been renamed Action for Sick Children (ASC) to reflect the needs of all children whether they be hospitalised or cared for in a community setting. The influence of all these people slowly brought a change to practice so that today families are actively encouraged to spend as much time as possible with their children.

Most importantly, more recent research (Carney *et al.*, 2003) has identified that children themselves view parental presence as a positive aspect of hospitalisation; unfortunately, Shields *et al.* (2004) suggest that the parental need to remain with their sick child, whatever their age, for 24 hours a day is not being met since there is a shortage of appropriate facilities.

**Table 2.3** Reactions displayed by the child experiencing parental separation
*(adapted from Robertson, 1958)*

| Stage | Reaction of the child separated from parents |
| --- | --- |
| Stage 1: Protest | • The child is grief-stricken, calling constantly for the parent(s). As the young child lives in the present, he/she may feel deserted by the parent(s).<br>• The child is likely to reject the healthcare professional and may become openly hostile. |
| Stage 2: Despair | • The child may sink into apparent depression, becoming quiet, apathetic and withdrawn, mourning for the lost parent(s).<br>• The child may adopt self-comforting behaviours, such as thumb-sucking, and may regress developmentally, for example in potty training, play activities or language.<br>• The child may exhibit behavioural difficulties and sleep problems.<br>• When parents visit, the child may become upset. |
| Stage 3: Denial | • The child no longer appears depressed and shows interest in the immediate surroundings.<br>• The child may now repress all feelings for the parent(s).<br>• If separation from the parent(s) is prolonged, he/she may settle into a new routine and way of life. This may lead to long-term emotional disturbances.<br>• The child may become the centre of the carers' attention |

---

**Activity**
*While it is generally accepted that it is extremely beneficial for a parent to remain with a sick child (whether they be hospitalised or in their own home), this can introduce other challenges. Take a moment to consider the difficulties that may be encountered by parents who decide to spend significant amounts of time with their sick child. What could be the implications of this decision for the whole family?*

You may have identified some of the following.

• Parents may feel obliged to stay with their child, particularly if they learn that this is the norm. This can lead to exhaustion and stress as the parent tries to juggle the family commitments from the bedside of a sick child. Parents have on occasions been heard to utter statements such as, 'I daren't leave her' (Teare and Smith, 2004, p. 32). Providing opportunities for parents to have a break may be crucial.

• There is evidence (Darbyshire, 1994; Teare and Smith, 2004) to suggest that healthcare professionals, especially nurses, expect parents to be with their sick child – if they decide not to be, this may provoke feelings of guilt and neglect. Good communication and negotiating skills will help to reassure parents that they do not have to be resident with their child.

- If the child is hospitalised, many children's wards do not include a wide range of resources, for instance parents may find themselves sleeping in a chair or, at best, a camp bed with little in the way of bed clothes. Toileting facilities may be limited with a lack of privacy, and parents may restrict their eating if they have to leave their child to visit the canteen.
- A parent of a hospitalised child may feel very isolated, particularly if they are being cared for in a cubicle. Boredom may be a problem with little diversion and few people to talk to. Introducing parents to others in a similar situation may help them to feel supported.
- If the child is being cared for at home, particularly if he or she has a condition that reduces mobility (such as a fractured shaft of femur), this also raises issues: the parent may find that they are confined to the house and unable to carry out the usual family commitments.
- In today's society, many parents work, and having to stay with a sick child could have significant work implications.
- Other family members, especially siblings, may feel that they are being ignored – this may be exacerbated if the sick child is being given treats. This can lead to behavioural problems, and parents may need advice about how to manage this situation and how to involve siblings in care.
- It is not usual for a parent to spend 24 hours a day constantly with a child, whatever their age.

It is clear that children of all ages need close family contact during their illness, but it is important that the other demands placed upon the family are recognised and that parents are encouraged to take breaks. In addition, families must not feel coerced into being resident with their child.


## FEELING SAFE

'Home' for families is frequently related to feelings of comfort, safety, familiarity, privacy and sanctuary (Darbyshire, 1994). These feelings may be lost if the environment is unfamiliar (for example during hospitalisation). In addition, parents may demonstrate considerable concern and anxiety for their sick child, frequently prompting a frightened and nervous demeanour. There is evidence to suggest that families need to trust healthcare professionals (Shields *et al.*, 2004) who are looking after their child. This leads to feelings of security and helps them to relax and to feel safe in the knowledge that appropriate care and treatment is being provided. A calm, empathetic approach that focuses upon the individual needs of the child and family is certainly beneficial. Similarly, it is important that families are able to build a rapport and therapeutic relationship with staff; so limiting the number of people who have contact with the child and parent may be appropriate – you may see that each child has a named nurse. It is essential to ensure that you appear reliable, well-informed and supportive to the family – this will facilitate the early discharge of the child (MacCallum *et al.*, 2001) and a return to normal family life. The provision of accurate information in language that the family will understand must also receive a high priority.

## WAITING

It is clear from the work of Teare and Smith (2004) that children and their parents may experience prolonged waiting times in relation to healthcare provision. This inevitably leads to frustration and annoyance. It is important to remember that families may have other commitments which require organisation (particularly in relation to other children and work) and, as a result, need to know what is going to happen to their child and when. Parents have little to occupy their minds when waiting in an outpatient's department, paediatric assessment unit or a ward. As a result, their focus will be firmly placed upon the clock and the number of hours that have passed since a member of staff last communicated to them about their child – it may well be this negative experience that they remember more than the positive ones. In recognition of this, the DH (2000) set a target in the NHS Plan that said that by December 2004 no one would spend longer than four hours in an accident and emergency department. The Report by the Comptroller and Auditor General (2004) stated that in the three months from April to June 2004 only 5.3% of patients stayed there that long, but suggested that there was a danger that focus could be placed upon the Government's target rather than concentrating on the completion of treatment. Even waiting for just three hours to be discharged home may seem an inordinately long time for a family.

---

**Activity**
*We all have to spend time waiting at moments in our lives. Think about how you could try to reduce the anxiety and frustration levels of families who are kept waiting.*

---

Perhaps you have thought about:

- being truthful to families. If there is likely to be a long wait, ensure that explanations are provided. Parents are likely to be far more understanding if they perceive that there is a clear reason for the delay.
- not ignoring parents. Revisit the family at frequent intervals to let them know that they have not been forgotten and to clarify progress.
- sitting with the child and family (time permitting). This will provide the opportunity for you to comfort them and to explain the proposed plan of events.
- ensuring that information is provided. Try to remember that the work environment is familiar territory to you, but families will need to know about

facilities such as toilets and the availability of food and drink. In addition, they may want assurance that their place in the queue will not be lost providing they inform staff of their whereabouts.

• keeping calm. You may well feel uncomfortable and embarrassed if a family has a long wait; maintaining a calm and professional manner is beneficial for everyone.

On a positive note, it is important to recognise that parents can be very impressed by the prompt and efficient service that their child receives.

## PARENTS AS PARTNERS IN CARE

Health care has undergone considerable change and development over the last decade, and parents are being actively encouraged not only to be involved in their children's care but also to take some control of it. Teare and Smith (2004) clearly identify that parents want to be involved in the care of their sick child; in addition, key documents, such as the Children Act (1989) and the more recent *National Service Framework for Children, Young People and Maternity Services* (DH and DfES, 2004), state that both the child and parents should be fully involved in decision-making processes.

When discussing the importance of working closely with families, the term 'family-centred care' is frequently used. This has been defined as:

the professional support of the child and family through a process of involvement, participation and partnership underpinned by empowerment and negotiation. (Smith *et al.*, 2002, p. 22)

Family-centred care is a concept that is widely respected; many healthcare professionals working with children and their families reflect its importance in their philosophies that are normally on display for all to see. It is clear from the above definition that family-centred care has many components; as a result, it is not always feasible to meet all aspects. In view of this, some clinical areas have chosen to focus on the achievement of a partnership approach in which families are encouraged to fully participate in the child's care. There can be no doubt that a lack of teamwork and communication between staff and families will lead to poor service provision for children (Hall and Elliman, 2003).

Lee (2004) does warn that there are usually two reasons why families participate in care, either because they want to or because they feel compelled to. One of the key aspects of working in partnership is negotiation, and it is imperative that families are not merely directed as to, or told, what tasks they should or can undertake. Good communication will ensure that families feel comfortable with the care role that they adopt for their sick child – it would be a mistake to assume that all parents want to participate in care activities, especially as they may never have had previous contact with the healthcare system.

---

**Activity**

*Take a moment to consider reasons why parents may be unable to, or may prefer not to, participate in their child's care.*

---

You may have thought about:

- tiredness/exhaustion;
- the possibility that the parent may know that the child does not want them to participate in physical care (e.g. a 13-year-old boy may not want his mother to help dress him);
- child-protection issues (please refer to Chapter 11);
- parental ill-health;
- lack of parental understanding and knowledge of child's illness and inability to participate in care – particularly immediately after diagnosis of the illness;
- the possibility that they simply may not want to;
- the fact that the child may have a close relationship with other people, such as grandparents.

Parental involvement in care is certainly beneficial, but it is essential to recognise that there may be good reasons for non-participation.


## CHILDREN AS PARTNERS IN CARE

There is sometimes a temptation to focus upon parental involvement in care; while this is important, it is also crucial to embrace the child's perspective and to encourage their active participation (The Children Act, 1989; DH and DfES, 2004). An anxiety that is sometimes voiced in relation to working in partnership with children is that they may not have the cognitive ability to make decisions (Dixon-Woods *et al.*, 1999). However, Flatman (2002) reminds us that recognising that children have a right to be listened to is not the same as giving them the responsibility for making decisions, but is involving them in care. In addition, children are continually undergoing a process of developmental growth and maturation that will eventually lead to adulthood and independence. It is therefore imperative that they are encouraged to take responsibility for their health. It is impossible to ascertain children's views about their health unless they are listened to and a partnership approach to care is adopted.

---

**Activity**

*Take a moment to think about how a partnership approach to care can be facilitated when working with children and their families.*

---

You may have identified the following.

- Recognition that the family (whatever its structure) is central to the child's life. An appreciation of the diversity of families within the UK will encourage you to consider who the child may have formed close relationships with (this is not always a genetic parent).
- Collaboration and discussion will facilitate identification of individual needs.
- Fostering an atmosphere that is respectful of individuals' views, cultural and religious beliefs. This will facilitate non-judgemental and non-discriminatory practice.
- The sharing of information with the child and family, that is at an appropriate level to facilitate full understanding. This should be provided in a supportive, caring manner that observes confidentiality (it is easy to forget that other people can hear through bedside curtains!).
- Recognition of the family's strengths. It is essential to remember that parents are experts in relation to knowledge about their child and they generally enjoy sharing this information. Acknowledging and using parents can not only facilitate good care, but also save time and help families to feel confident in their abilities and able to take control of their child's healthcare needs.
- Encouraging the family to spend as much time with the child as they want and explaining the activities that they can become involved in (these will be very diverse and may include simple day-to-day tasks, such as washing and dressing, or may be more complex depending upon the child's illness and the willingness of the family to learn new aspects of care). Likewise, the child should be encouraged to undertake personal self-care activities that are appropriate to their age and stage of development.
- Understanding the developmental and emotional needs of children.

A discussion about working in partnership with families would not be complete without mention of the diversity of cultures within the UK. In Britain, three million people (5.5 % of the population) are from black or ethnic minority groups, the majority of whom live in large towns or cities (Watt and Norton, 2004). In addition, the DH (2000b, p. 38) has indicated that children below 15 years of age form '33% of black and ethnic minority communities compared to 19% in white communities'. As a result, it is imperative that the care offered to children and their families is not only individually planned but also considers cultural needs.

Giger and Davidhizar offer a clear and detailed definition of culture:

> [Culture is a] behavioural response that develops over time as a result of imprinting the mind through social and religious structures and intellectual and artistic manifestations. (Giger and Davidhizar, 1995, p. 3)

This definition is not to be confused with other relating concepts, such as race, which refers to the particular physical characteristics of a group of people (Giger and Davidhizar, 1999) or ethnicity which relates to the 'cultural practices and attitudes that characterise a given group of people' (Watt and Norton, 2004, p. 38).

There is a danger that if the care provided is not sensitive to the cultural needs of the family, the child may find the hospital environment particularly alien and disturbing; this could potentially affect the physical and psychological well-being of the child. For some time there have been strong suggestions that care should embrace the cultural needs of patients (Leininger, 1991; McGee, 1994; Chevannes, 2002) and it is something that has been advocated within recent Government documents (DH and DfES, 2004).

---

**Activity**
*Think of why it may be beneficial to take the cultural needs of the child and family into consideration.*

---

You may have considered the following points.

- The extended family may be extremely important and a wide number of people may be actively involved in child care. However, it has been suggested that 'the involvement of the extended family in family-centred care remains non-existent' (Ochieng, 2003, p. 124).
- Some family members may not be fluent in the English language, necessitating good support from interpreters. Casey (1995) comments that cultural differences and language difficulties may exclude parents, and she continues by saying that families who do not speak English are less likely to participate in care.
- The culturally perceived cause of an illness may be significant in determining the family's response to the sick child.
- The expectations for survival of the child may affect the family's attitude to immediate and long-term care.
- The future social roles that are thought to be appropriate for the disabled or chronically ill child may affect the resources and time that a family is willing to apply to health care and education.

In addition, Watt and Norton (2004) suggest some points of good practice (Table 2.4).

**Table 2.4** Points of good practice when working with children and families from different cultures *(adapted from Watt and Norton, 2004)*

- Make the effort to learn key words or phrases.
- Remember that facial gestures, body posture and voice intonation will communicate more than the spoken word.
- Get down to the child's eye level, but don't be anxious if he/she avoids eye contact – this could be a sign of respect.
- Speak clearly, but avoid shouting.
- Wherever possible, use trained interpreters – family members may be selective about the information that they pass on, particularly if it is of a sensitive nature.

Clearly, it is not practicable to learn about the whole range of cultures that exist within the UK. First of all, there are so many that it would not be feasible to cover them all; secondly, there appears to be no evidence to suggest that knowledge of one culture helps someone to provide better care for a child of another; thirdly, it portrays sensitivity to individual cultures in a simplistic manner.

---

**Activity**

*How do you think that an appreciation of differing cultures can be facilitated?*

---

Have you considered:

- an appreciation of your own culture? We all feel an affiliation to a particular culture; by considering how important this is to us will help us to understand the value of culture to others.
- a desire to facilitate effective communication? This may necessitate the use of a range of alternative strategies.
- *everyone's* cultural needs?
- acknowledging that there are differing perceptions of health, illness and treatment across cultures?
- a willingness to practise in an anti-discriminatory manner that respects people of all cultures?

All of the above points will facilitate an appreciation of cultural diversity and the impact that it has on a child and family's perception of their health needs. This can only further enhance care.


## CONCLUSION

There is no doubt that working with children and their families can be emotionally and physically challenging. You may encounter difficult and demanding situations that require you to reflect upon your own beliefs and personal attributes; however, you should feel stimulated and valued as part of a multidisciplinary team. Children are the future of our society and deserve the best possible care – enjoy providing it!


## REFERENCES

Bernardes J (1997) *Family studies: An introduction.* London: Routledge.

Carling A (2002) Family policy, social theory and the state. In: Carling A, Duncan S and Edwards R (eds) *Analysing Families: Morality and rationality in policy and practice.* London: Routledge.

Carney T, Murphy S, McClure J, Bishop E, Kerr C, Parker J *et al.* (2003) Children's views of hospitalisation: An exploratory study of data collection. *Journal of Child Health Care* 7(1), 27–40.

Carter B (2004) Editorial: If I have to say it one more time, I swear I'm gonna kill someone. *Journal of Child Health Care* 8(3), 178–179.

Casey A (1995) Partnership nursing: influences on involvement of informal carers. *Journal of Advanced Nursing* 22(6), 1058–1062.

Chevannes M (2002) Issues in educating health professionals to meet the diverse needs of patients and other service users from ethnic minority groups. *Journal of Advanced Nursing* 39(3), 290–298.

Crawford DA (2002) Keep the focus on the family. *Journal of Child Health Care* 6(2), 133–146.

Darbyshire P (1994) *Living with a sick child in hospital: The experiences of parents and nurses.* London: Chapman & Hall.

Department of Health (DH) (2000a) *The NHS plan: A plan for investment – A plan for reform.* London: DH/DfES.

Department of Health (DH) (2000b) *Assessing children in need and their families.* London: DH.

Department of Health (DH) (2002) *National Service Framework for Children*: London: DH.

Department of Health and Department for Education and Skills (DH/DfES) (2004) *National Service Framework for Children, Young People and Maternity Services.* London: DH.

Dixon-Woods M, Young B and Heney D (1999) Partnerships with children. *British Medical Journal* 319(7212), 778–780.

European Parliament, Council of the European Union and European Commission (2000) *Charter of fundamental rights of the European Union.* Official Journal of the European Communities C364, Nice.

Flatman D (2002) Consulting with children: are we listening? *Paediatric Nursing* 14(7), 28–31.

Giger JL and Davidhizar RE (1995) *Transcultural Nursing: Assessment and intervention* (2nd edn). St Louis: Mosby.

Giger JN and Davidhizar RE (1999) *Transcultural Nursing: Assessment and intervention* (3rd edn). St Louis: Mosby.

Hall DMB and Elliman D (eds) (2003) *Health for all Children* (4th edn). Oxford: Oxford University Press.

Lee P (2004) Family involvement: Are we asking too much? *Paediatric Nursing* 16(10), 37–41.

Leininger M (1991) *Culture Care Diversity and Universality: A theory of nursing.* New York: National League for Nursing.

Lindsay B (2003) A 2-year-old goes to hospital: A 50th anniversary reappraisal of the impact of James Robertson's film. *Journal of Child Health Care* 7(1), 17–26.

Lowton K (2002) Parents and partners: Lay carers' perceptions of their role in the treatment and care of adults with cystic fibrosis. *Journal of Advanced Nursing* 39(2), 174–181.

MacCallum PL, MacRae DL, Sukerman S and MacRae E (2001) Ambulatory adenoidotonsillectomy in children less than 5 years of age. *Journal of Otolaryngology* 30(2), 75–78.

McGee P (1994) Culturally sensitive and culturally comprehensive care. *British Journal of Nursing* 3(15), 789–792.

Ochieng BMN (2003) Minority ethnic families and family-centred care. *Journal of Child Health Care* 7(2), 123–132.

Report by the Comptroller and Auditor General (2004) *Improving Emergency Care in England.* Report by the Comptroller and Auditor General. HC 1075 Session 2003–2004: 13 October 2004. London: TSO.

Richards M (1995) Family relationships: Relationships within families. *The Psychologist* 8(2), 70–72.

Robertson J (1958) *Young Children in Hospital.* London: Tavistock Publications.

Rutherford D (1998) Children's relationships. In: Taylor J and Woods M (eds) *Early Childhood Studies: An holistic introduction.* London: Arnold Publishers.

Shields L, Hunter J and Hall J (2004) Parents' and staff's perceptions of parental needs during a child's admission to hospital: An English perspective. *Journal of Child Health Care* 8(1), 9–33.

Smith L, Coleman V and Bradshaw M (2002) *Family-centred care: Concept, theory and practice.* Basingstoke: Palgrave.

Taylor J and Müller D (1994) *Nursing Adolescents: Research and psychological perspectives.* Oxford: Blackwell Science.

Taylor P, Richardson J, Yeo A, Marsh I, Trobe K and Pilkington A (1995) *Sociology in Focus.* London: Causeway Press.

Teare J and Smith J (2004) Using focus groups to explore the views of parents whose children are in hospital. *Paediatric Nursing* 16(5), 30–35.

United Nations (1998) *Fiftieth Anniversary of the Universal Declaration of Human Rights.* Geneva: United Nations.

United Nations Children's Fund (UNICEF) (2001) *A league table of births in rich nations.* Innocenti Report Card No 3. Italy: UNICEF, Florence.

Watt S and Norton D (2004) Culture, ethnicity, race: What's the difference? *Paediatric Nursing* 16(8), 37–42.

# 3 Communicating with Children and Families

**P. VICKERS**

## INTRODUCTION

We all communicate. Just by looking at somebody we communicate. We point, we gesture and, perhaps most importantly, we use verbal sounds, or language. Not just humans communicate, but all animals as well, including single-cell animals such as the amoeba and bacteria. Even the cells of our bodies communicate with each other. This chapter considers ways in which the healthcare worker can communicate with children and their families who come under their care. It will not cover every means of communication, for example 'signing', which is a specialised method; rather, it will consider the ways in which children communicate as part of their normal development. Chapter 8 also considers communication; that chapter discusses how children communicate when playing.

---

**Activity**
*Before beginning this chapter, just write down what you think is meant by 'communication'?*

---

You may have looked in your dictionary for the meaning. For example, in the *Chambers Dictionary* (1998), the verb 'to communicate' is defined as 'to succeed in conveying one's meaning to others'.

The *Concise Oxford Dictionary* (Allen, 1993) gives several definitions for communication, including:

- 'the act of imparting, especially news';
- 'the information, etc. communicated';
- 'a means of connecting different places, such as a door, passage, road, or railway';
- 'social intercourse';
- 'the science and practice of transmitting information especially by electronic or mechanical means';
- 'a paper read to a learned society'.

---

*Caring for Children and Families*. Edited by I. Peate and L. Whiting
© 2006 John Wiley & Sons Ltd

Did any of the things that you noted match with any of the definitions above?

Communication is meant to convey information from one person to another person or to other people (or, indeed, to animals). This information can be conveyed by both verbal and non-verbal means. Much of the information conveyed by babies and very young children is by non-verbal means, for example by pointing and by gesturing, by posture and by facial expressions. Non-verbal communication allows us to some degree to get others to do what we want for us. Non-verbal communication is also very good at revealing our attitudes, for example our like or dislike of something or someone, how interested we are in something or someone and even our understanding of what someone else is saying.

However, purely non-verbal communication does not have the precision that allows us to communicate more abstract thoughts, behaviours and wishes/needs, nor to communicate the scale of time and space. For this we need oral communication in the form of language, because non-verbal gestures and facial expressions can only operate in the here and now. With language, which includes both vocabulary and grammar, we are able to discuss things from the past as well as things for the future. We can also explain things that are happening or that have to be done. With language comes imagination – language is creative. All that is necessary is that the speaker and the listener understand the words and the rules of grammar in the same way. It also means that the listener has to concentrate on what the speaker is saying, and the speaker has to concentrate to be reassured that the listener is following and understanding what is being said.

According to Reynolds (1997), the best-known model of communication is the one devised by Shannon and Weaver (1949), which is a simple linear model that is easily understood. The model has five main parts:

- a source of information – this is where the message is produced;
- a transmitter – this is where the message is encoded;
- a channel – this carries a signal to where it's going;
- a receiver – this is where the message is decoded;
- a destination – this is where the message finally ends up.

All this may seem quite complicated, but if you think about what you have learnt so far in this chapter, and then integrate it with Shannon and Weaver's (1949) model, you can see the framework in action:

- Information source – the author of this chapter;
- Transmitter – the author has used written words and language to encode the message;
- Channel – this book that you have bought or borrowed and are reading;
- Receiver – your eyes, optic nerve, brain;
- Destination – you, your brain and your understanding.

Think of any conversation that you have had with somebody recently. Try to apply that conversation to the above model. You can see that it makes good sense and fits in with communication. However, Reynolds (1997) concludes that although this transmission model has good points it is not an accurate reflection of the complex nature of communication. She says that it does not allow for:

- the construction of meaning;
- the context of the communication;
- the purpose of the communication;
- the relationship between the two parties involved, namely the information source and the destination;
- the influence of the chosen medium.

These are all essential parts of communication, which is a complex and interactive process that relies upon the active participation of both the sender and receiver. Although the sender is the person who decides the content of the communication, and the form in which it is going to be communicated, the receiver of the communication is just as important because without a receiver the communication may just as well not exist.

Buckley (2003) emphasises that human communication involves a combination and interplay of skills, including:

- language (highly individual to societies and individuals);
- mental processes (e.g. finding meaning in other people's speech/vocabulary);
- physical movements (e.g. posture, gesturing with hands/fingers/head and facial expressions).

## WHY COMMUNICATE?

We communicate because we are social animals, and, if we are to easily interact, we need good communication skills. We also need to develop our communication skills in order to have some control over our social and emotional worlds and to relate to others (Buckley, 2003). As far as children are concerned, they need to be able to communicate their needs because they are so dependent upon adults. As they grow and develop, communication gives them access to education, and later to work. In addition, these developing communication skills allow children to take part in all other areas of life, including the world of leisure and, probably most important of all, relationships (Buckley, 2003). As the Department for Education and Skills (DfES) states in its publication *Common Code of Skills and Knowledge for the Children's Workforce* (2005, p. 6), 'Good communication is central to working with children, young people, their parents and carers.'

## COMMUNICATING WITH CHILDREN

One of the essential things to remember when communicating with children is that what an adult thinks the aim of the communication is may not necessarily be the same as what the child thinks. Sometimes, the meanings may be completely the opposite. One of the major reasons for this is that the adult communicating a message may include complicated and sometimes abstract concepts that are far beyond the understanding and reasoning ability of the child. Communication is not just about speaking; it involves such activities as listening, questioning and understanding, as well as responding to what is being communicated. It is not just about language or the words that are used; there are many other factors involved, such as tone of voice and manner of speaking, as well as body language. Perhaps most important of all, is the effectiveness of the listening process (DfES, 2005). This facilitates the building of trust between the child, the parents and the carers. The DfES (2005) details two key requirements when carers need to communicate and engage with children and their families. First of all, it says that in order to build a rapport with children, young people and their families it is essential to demonstrate understanding, respect and honesty – while the second requirement is continuity in relationships. Both of these help to promote engagement and communication.

So how do children communicate? Like adults, they communicate in a variety of ways, but unlike adults these different ways are not extras, but rather are essentials. The reason for this is that until children develop the skills and vocabulary for communication by speech, they have to communicate by whatever means they can.

Initially, newborn babies communicate mainly by crying and posture/movement. Their mothers and fathers, as well as their carers, very quickly learn to recognise the different types of cries and what each individual posture and movement means. In fact, communication commences the moment a baby is born. Babies and their parents develop their own special relationships by developing their own unique communication patterns. This means that it is often difficult for an outsider to understand and be able to meet a baby's need. So if you are working with a baby and parent, it is a good idea, before becoming involved, to spend some time observing how the baby and the parent communicate. This will allow you to participate in the care of the baby and to build a relationship with the family. There are, in addition, some basic rules to facilitate communication with babies.

**Activity**
*If you were asked to look after baby Jasmine whose parents were not present and you have not had an opportunity to observe the family interaction, how would you communicate with Jasmine so that you could meet all of her basic and social needs?*

Have you thought about the following.

- Observing how Jasmine cries and moves, as well as the postures she maintains when requiring a basic need to be taken care of, for example feeding or nappy changing. You will soon pick up on these visual and aural clues and be able to quickly meet her needs.
- Making and maintaining eye contact whenever you are with Jasmine and she is awake.
- Communicating your feelings for Jasmine by the way in which you make physical contact, i.e. holding, cuddling and stroking. This, of course, can be a double-edged sword, because of the physical contact, Jasmine will soon pick up on your mood and this could affect her. For example, if you are tense, unhappy or in a hurry, Jasmine may become miserable. However, if you are in a relaxed and happy frame of mind, Jasmine should also become relaxed and happy.
- Constantly talking, murmuring or singing to Jasmine whenever you are doing any care, or just holding/cuddling her, or playing with her. As long as the noises you are making are warm and comforting, Jasmine will be more relaxed. However, if there is an edge to your voice, or your tone is harsh, then Jasmine may become unsettled and unhappy.
- Having fun with Jasmine, you will discover lots of ways in which you can communicate with her – touch, facial expressions, eye contact, words and sounds, and silly games such as peek-a-boo.
- Connecting and communicating with Jasmine to help feelings of security will also help to enhance learning.

## COMMUNICATING THROUGH LANGUAGE

By the time a baby becomes a toddler, he or she is beginning to speak, rather than communicating by crying and other non-verbal means. However, what is speech? According to Buckley (2003), speech is the use of sounds in order to express language, and as Golinkoff and Hirsh-Pasek (1999, p. 1) state, 'Communicating through language is the crowning achievement of the human species . . . within every infant lies the potential to learn a language.'

Language is not just about speech. There are other forms of language expression. For example, there is writing, sign language and other visual means of communication, such as drawing and painting.

The toddler has gone through many stages in developing their ability to speak. For example, at about four months of age, a baby will coo and gurgle with great confidence. Although this may seem meaningless to the adult, the baby is physically preparing for speech. Speech occurs as a result of a series of intricate muscular movements in and around the mouth, and involves the lips, the tongue, the soft palate and the roof of the mouth, the pharynx and the jaw. In actual fact, the baby has been preparing to speak since birth as the act of suckling at the breast or bottle helps to push the jaw forward and to strengthen the jaw muscles.

However, speech is not only a physical manifestation – there has to be thought, knowledge and structure behind speech. All this comes about through the baby's exploration of her or his environment as well as through interactions between the baby and others. The growth of language and communication skills requires this partnership between the child and the environment; however, the most significant partner is the adult carer because both the child and the adult need to work together to achieve mutual understanding. Initially, this mutual understanding occurs non-verbally, but later it occurs through language (Jarvis and Lamb, 2001). This process is essential not only for the development of communication skills but also for the child's emotional development and well-being (Goldschmied and Selleck, 1996). So all the time that the baby is babbling, they are actually learning how to move their lips and tongue to replicate the sounds heard around them.

By the time the baby has become a toddler, he or she understands far more than he or she can actually say. This situation is similar to someone learning a foreign language. If you are having French lessons, your understanding of what is being said to you in that language is greater than your ability to speak that language. So it is with our toddler – he or she can understand simple words, commands, sentences and even concepts without being able to put them into words. It has been found that in the early stages of development a particular word or phrase can only be understood when it is spoken in a particular context that is understood by the child or when accompanied by a particular gesture (Pease *et al.*, 1989). So, at this stage in their development, children's ability to understand more words than they can say is based upon their interpretation of the context of the word and the use of non-verbal strategies (Buckley, 2003).

There are a number of useful tips when communicating with young children. It is important to speak slowly and clearly to the toddler and to give them plenty of time to try to think of the words that they need to express themselves. In addition, it may be necessary to repeat any instructions, using simple phrases and ensuring that the toddler has understood what you have been saying. Remember that the toddler is easily frightened by strangers; so, as with the baby, it is important to use lots of smiles, plenty of eye contact and relaxed and friendly/comforting body language, particularly if the parents are not present.

Toddlers express themselves not only with language, however basic it may be, but also through play. Children spend a great deal of their time playing, either with others or on their own. Play has been recognised as essential for normal growth and development (Chambers, 1993); toddlers' play reflects their developing understanding about the world and their symbolic understanding and conceptual organisation (Buckley, 2003). Types of play behaviours have been found to accompany particular developments in communication (Paul, 1995; Buckley, 2003). For example, at 14 months, children may make a pretence of undertaking simple activities, such as brushing their hair or talking on a toy telephone (Buckley, 2003). These acts are linked to the development of language; at this age, children are handling objects in the way that they are actually used, and this reflects the child's developing ability to organise objects. Family members and carers of children label things according to how the children appear to organise them, and this helps the child to know how words relate to objects (Buckley, 2003). These isolated simple activities are quickly followed by simple sequenced events, such as pretending to feed their dolls or having pretend tea parties. This again shadows their language development, in that they start to link words rather than using just one word.

Throughout this time when the child is a toddler and exploring her or his environment, symbolic development is occurring gradually. Between the ages of 10 and 24 months, children progress from the stage of communicating through conventional signals (mainly vocal sounds and gestures) to communicating through symbols, that is words and focused, representational gestures (Camaioni *et al.*, 2003). In this context, a symbol is something that 'stands for something else, such as a toy cup or a picture of a cup which can represent the concept of a cup' (Buckley, 2003, pp. 53–54). Contextual factors (the realism of toys and the play situation) have a great impact on symbolic play (Umek and Musek, 2001). According to Cooper *et al.*, (1978) cited in Buckley (2003), symbolic understanding of the child will gradually increase so that eventually he or she is able to link what are increasingly arbitrary representations of objects/events to concepts that are relevant to the child's experiences and environment. The carer/parent can often pick up on what the child is trying to say by observing the child at play. A child may often only be able to express needs, wants, fears or emotions through play. It is then up to the carer, whether they be a family member or professional, to identify the clues that come from the child's play.

By the time children are 4 years of age, they are able to:

- understand sentences with up to six separate pieces of information;
- follow and participate in many different conversations;
- understand lengthy instructions, such as may be given in the nursery classroom (Buckley, 2003);
- understand basic grammatical structures (Tager-Flusberg, 1989, cited in Buckley, 2003).

Children, by the age of 5 years, are able to follow stories and are also able to respond appropriately to complex questions (Buckley, 2003). So during these years, with their continuous development, in order to develop an understanding of language, children have a need for conversations. Conversations now give them many opportunities not only to get their own meanings and intentions across to others but also to interpret the intentions of others. Thus, the adult now finds it easier to communicate with children. Indeed, during these years, children's abilities to hold conversations progress to include topics that are initiated by other people, not just themselves. In particular, they are able to take turns in speaking.

As well as the conversations changing (becoming longer and more cooperative), children continue to communicate using play. However, the major change with play is that it becomes an increasingly social activity with a greater reliance on effective interaction and language skills (Buckley, 2003). Play has now become sophisticated enough to include the development of:

- abstract thought;
- peer relationships and friendships;
- the child's understanding of the world and social relationships through the medium of the physical activity inherent within play at this age;
- narrative skills – such as the organising of real or imagined events (Garvey, 1977; Hetherington and Parke, 1986, cited in Buckley, 2003).

## COMMUNICATING THROUGH PLAY

Children will use play as a medium for expressing themselves or for communicating with others (Chambers, 1993). When trying to understand what a child is trying to communicate through play, it is essential to remember that all objects can stand for other different things, just as people can take on roles that they would not ordinarily play in real life (Golinkoff and Hirsh-Pasek, 1999).

Some of the play that children take part in can be partly verbal, and this does sometimes reveal children's sensitivity to the roles that people take on when around them. They are also sensitive to the way that people within their sphere of experience actually communicate verbally (Golinkoff and Hirsch-Pasek, 1999). For instance, toddlers have the ability to duplicate the way that adults talk to them and to babies. When toddlers play the role of 'mother', they often increase the pitch of their voices and talk in shorter sentences and ask their 'baby' questions about their physical needs. There was one memorable interview that was recorded during research looking at the experiences of children who had been isolated for health reasons for many months at a young age (Vickers, 1999). In it, the father of a girl, Aisha, who had been cared for in an isolation cubicle from 3 months of age until she was almost 3 years old, was asked how Aisha (then nearly 5 years old) related with other children of her age. He replied, 'She has a very adult relationship to other children. I think she's been so used to being treated by adults, and talked to by adults, that she employs exactly the same treatment with other children. She talks in sound bites. She asks them how they are, what their names are. A bit like a doctor does – and then goes off and does something else!' (Vickers, 1999, p. 352).

Children's pretend play is very often the origin of their earliest narrative (Golinkoff and Hirsh-Pasek, 1999). They tell a story with their play. This story may be based upon something that they have seen that demonstrates what they're feeling at that moment. For example, children who are suddenly thrust into a strange environment, such as a hospital ward or a nursery, may use play to work through their feelings and fears, while at the same time they may be letting the adults know that they have concerns about where they are (Chambers, 1993). If parents leave their child in the care of adults who are strangers, he or she may use play to work through feelings of abandonment. The astute and empathetic adult will be able to recognise this play as a form of communication, will be able to join in the play and so gain her or his trust.

Adults are important characters within children's play. When adults play roles within children's play, they open a door to another play world that children can then enter (Lindqvist, 2001). During this time of play, the adults will use verbal as well as physical and tactile communications. This adult talk provides a structure for the child's actions, which in turn helps to set up the pretend reality that allows him or her to communicate meaningfully through play. In addition, the child is able to see how useful language can be for transforming situations and for communicating (Golinkoff and Hirsh-Pasek, 1999). Another very important aspect of adults becoming involved in children's play is that they tend to talk much more about motivations and beliefs than children; this gives children insights into how language can be used to talk about others' thoughts and feelings, thus helping them to progress from completely self-centred babies to more thoughtful and well-rounded children.

During pretend play, children are able to adopt roles that reflect people other than themselves, for example mother, father, teacher, cowboy or anybody they have come into contact with in reality or on the television or cinema screen. This allows play to become more complex and for children to take part in social play within groups.

At about 5 years of age, communication skills are fundamental to the development of play. As Buckley (2003, p. 121) points out, 'As pretend play moves increasingly towards becoming a social activity that is based on ideas, the need for social interaction skills and the ability to understand and communicate ideas becomes greater.' With pretend play moving increasingly towards a social activity, communicative functions need to be expressed very clearly and cooperatively. This includes making plans, 'deciding what role each child will play', the objective of the play and the pretend environment. Perhaps one of the greatest changes that comes about with social play is that children need to be flexible not only in their actions but in their communication skills, because the focus of their play and each individual child's role may alter.

However, if children find themselves in a strange environment, such as a school or a hospital ward, they may well regress, and conversation becomes a harder activity. Communication with children in this situation may well return to the same forms as those used with toddlers.

## COMMUNICATING BY DRAWING*

Children at any age have yet another means of communicating, namely by drawings/paintings and other forms of visual artistic expression. Children love to draw, and learn this skill before they can write – even if it only appears to the outsider as a series of scribbles, to the child it will have much meaning (Oster and Gould, 1987). One of the first people to use art as an aid to communication with children was DiLeo. In 1970 he stated that a child draws what he or she knows, not what he or she sees. Later, in 1983, DiLeo wrote that there were three groups of people whose art may be regarded as genuine and authentic because it is generally free from cultural intrusion. One of those groups, he says, is composed of young children who still cling to a vision from 'an innocent eye'. Incidentally, the other two groups were said to be the 'mentally subnormal' and ' those we call mad' (DiLeo, 1983, p. 175).

Johnson (1990) argues that children may speak to us more clearly and openly through their drawings than they are willing, or able, to do verbally. Kelley (1985) also found that children were able to express their experiences and feelings in drawing and painting, even though they were unable to verbalise them. She found that the act of drawing decreased children's anxiety because they could lose themselves in the actual manual activity. Thomas and Silk (1990) take this further and point out that the child's drawing is coloured by his or her feelings. Veltman and Browne (2001) agree and say, 'This is what makes drawings, potentially, so significant as expressions of personality, and useful for the identification of emotional problems in children' (p. 251).

Even prior to DiLeo, the narrative and emotional value of using children's drawings as aids to communication had been identified. Hulse (1952) writes that having a child draw his family actually provides very useful information about how that child perceives and interacts with his family. This is important because directly questioning a child about their view of their family, or any significant experience, is rarely an effective way of uncovering that child's feelings (Veltman and Browne, 2001).

Although children from an early age do possess varying degrees of confidence with spoken and oral language, they often prefer to express and communicate what is going on in their world through non-verbal expressions. That said, according to Walker (1998, p. 263), 'the use of play and art can facilitate exploration, problem solving, growth and understanding emotionally and cognitively [of] the self and the world'. Walker (1998) suggests that many adults are confused by, and unfamiliar with, children's non-verbal communication. In particular, they do not understand the importance to the child of his or her play, games, stories and art. There is a tremendous desire on the part of the adult for the child to communicate primarily through spoken and written language from as early an age as possible. This is commonly seen in parents who may state 'my child spoke at 12 months', 'but mine spoke at 10 months',

*All names used in this section are pseudonyms.

for example. This kind of competitiveness does not help the child to creatively and fluently express himself/herself in a way with which he or she is comfortable. As Walker (1998, p. 263) states, this 'keeps children's knowledge in the margins if children are unable to express themselves well verbally'.

Much of the work with children and art has been done by art therapists and psychotherapists. One such example was discussed by Linesch (2002), an American therapist who, with her class of students, took an art session with a group of children from the kindergarten to the eighth grade (from 4 to 14 years) the day after the destruction of the World Trade Center on September 11th 2001. They had been reassured that the children were unscathed by the terrorism and, since the parents had been asked not to allow the children to watch the television, the children were unaware of details. However, despite this, Linesch writes, 'the art that emerged spoke from aching hearts and minds to attending hearts and minds' (p. 156). The children all drew images from the previous day's destruction – some of them quite horrific, but this was the way in which the children tried to make sense of what had occurred, and tried to work through their feelings about it.

Another example of the power of children's art and the way that it allows children to express their thoughts, feelings and turmoils was seen recently in Berlin, Germany (Paterson, 2005). An exhibition of school children's art from the Nazi era illustrated in detail what adolescents chose – or were ordered – to draw in the Third Reich while they attended art classes at Munich schools during the 1930s and early 1940s. Again, the images are very powerful, but, while those of the American children in 2001 demonstrated horror, uncertainty and fear, these paintings in Germany from over 60 years ago showed a glorification of German might and brutality.

There are several sources which can help the non-therapist to use children's drawings as an aid to communicating with the children, and in 1987 Oster and Gould combined what had been published to date and made lists of what to look for. When trying to communicate with a child using their drawings, it is important to be there with them and to discuss what they are doing. For example, what may be an unformed blob to the adult may well be a representation of a very important person to the child. The following drawings will demonstrate what can be achieved by way of communicating using drawings. These pictures drawn by English and German children who had been nursed in isolation cubicles were produced as part of a major research study (Vickers, 1999). Initially, during interviews with the families of the children, many of them said that their children were unaffected by their isolation as babies and toddlers. However, when the children were asked to draw pictures of themselves, their families, their hobbies and their house a different image started to emerge.

The first picture (Figure 3.1) is a self-portrait of Wilhelm, a German boy who was almost 10 years old at the time of the research. When asked to draw himself, he produced an image of a child vomiting bright red blood. Once I had discussed this with him and his family, they admitted that he was often

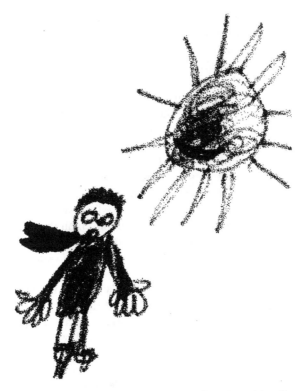

**Figure 3.1** Self-portrait by Wilhelm (vomiting blood).

unhappy, had changed his school and that he had few friends. Without Wilhelm's drawing, a totally false picture of his situation may have been accepted by the health professionals, and also possibly his parents.

The picture in Figure 3.2 was drawn by Thomas, an English boy who was almost 7 years old at the time and shows what Thomas thinks about his family situation. His parents were not married, and his father, following arguments and disagreements, often left the family home to return months later. This obviously upset Thomas because, when asked to draw his family, he identified himself as the one who managed to keep the family together. He felt that, if he weren't there, his parents would break up completely.

The next four drawings (Figures 3.3, 3.4, 3.5 and 3.6) are by Theresia, a 5-year-old German girl. As a result of her illness and successful treatment, Theresia had very fine, scanty hair and her skin was mottled. She drew herself, her mother and her sister all the same with scanty hair and mottled skin, but her father with relatively unmarked skin. She did not want to be different from everybody else and, as she could not change, wanted all the other females in the family to be like her. Her father was allowed to be 'normal'; in fact, it almost seems as if the blemishes have fallen off her father's face and are lying

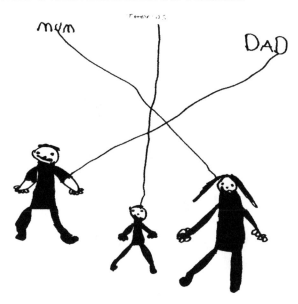

**Figure 3.2** Thomas and his parents (Thomas is the figure in the middle).

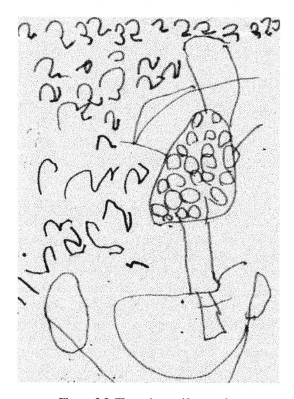

**Figure 3.3** Theresia – self-portrait.

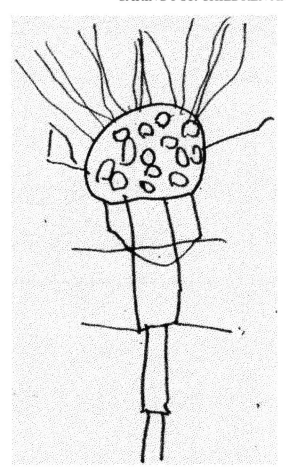

**Figure 3.4** Theresia – sister.

around his feet. Following these drawings, Theresia's elder sister did tell her mother that other children called Theresia names such as 'baldy', and this upset her. Her mother did not realise how much it affected Theresia, because she had always told her that she was perfectly normal and as beautiful as her sister.

One of the defining themes that came out of this research was that of 'alienation' – alienation of the child from the family and vice versa, alienation of the parents from the extended family, alienation of the parents from each other, alienation of the children from their peers and even alienation of the family from their society. This theme was first identified from the children's drawings, was then noticed in their lists of favourite activities and definitively confirmed by the children's families and schoolteachers.

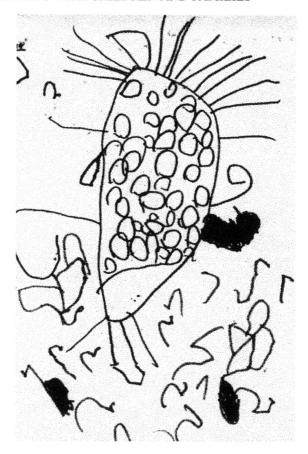

**Figure 3.5** Theresia – mother.

Seen in Figure 3.7 is John (9-year-old English boy) running away from his family. Underneath the drawing of himself, John has written 'Me: speeding', while under the drawing of his mother he has written 'Mam: holding Sheila' and beneath his father 'Dad: looking at Sheila'. His mother is saying 'Be quiet, Sheila' (Sheila is John's baby sister, who was, and always had been, perfectly healthy).

The next drawing (Figure 3.8) shows Henry (an English boy who was nearly 13 years old), who, when he was asked to draw something he enjoyed doing, showed himself sailing with the scouts. However, he was with his scoutmaster, not with his peers.

Henry also drew himself (Figure 3.9) sitting at home doing mathematics (again in response to being asked to draw what he liked doing best). This is a very solitary occupation.

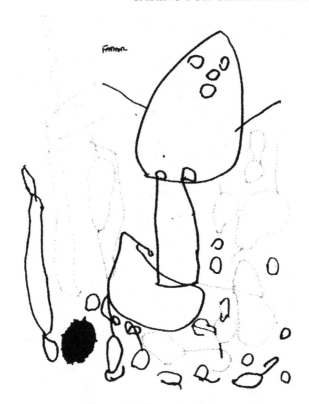

**Figure 3.6** Theresia – father.

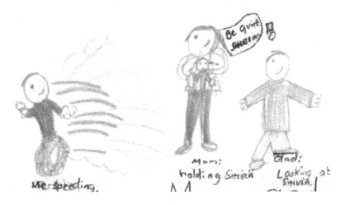

**Figure 3.7** John – running away from his family.

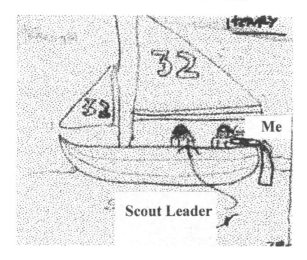

**Figure 3.8** Henry – 'my favourite hobbies.' (1).

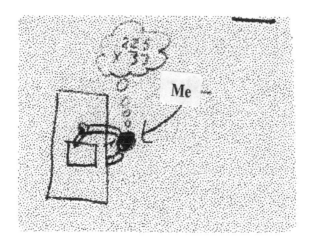

**Figure 3.9** Henry – 'my favourite hobbies' (2).

Franz (a 12-and-a-half-year-old Swiss boy) drew himself standing apart from his parents, looking suspiciously at them (Figure 3.10). Of note here is Franz's arm across his body – a very defensive posture. The other things to note are the 'talons' that his mother has; in the original coloured drawing they were a bright scarlet colour. According to Oster and Gould (1987), the sideways glances of Franz and his parents are a sign of suspicion and paranoid tendencies.

Finally, what did the children think of doctors and nurses? Birgit (a 6-and-a-half-year-old German girl) decided that she wanted to draw the interviewer.

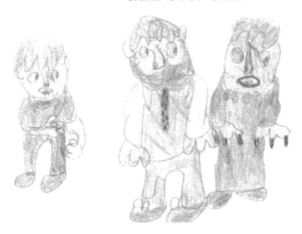

**Figure 3.10** Franz – with his parents.

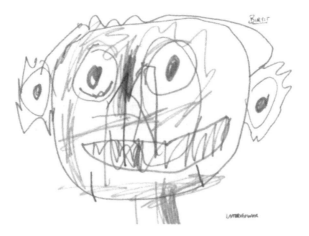

**Figure 3.11** Birgit – a drawing of the interviewer.

She had only just met him, but he must have represented all the people who had stuck needles into her, and generally made life difficult and painful for her (as she perceived it). This drawing (Figure 3.11) carries all the anger, frustration and hatred of the health professionals in it, and has not lost anything from being reproduced in black and white. The very sharp, pointed teeth are an indication of aggression, while overemphasis on the ears equates to a degree of suspiciousness and fear, as do the staring eyes.

As can be seen, drawings have become an excellent source for expressing present concerns and conflicts. Although the examples above are of people, art therapists often ask children to draw other things, particularly the house that they live in or a tree (Oster and Gould, 1987). A tree is a very useful object because it is impersonal and so children may feel that they can transfer their own feelings onto the tree as it is safe to do so. This chapter does not aim to investigate the therapeutic aspects of children's drawings; it is merely intended to demonstrate that it is possible to use drawings as a way of entering the child's world and stimulating communication.

## COMMUNICATING WITH ADOLESCENTS

Adolescents inhabit that awkward time between childhood and adulthood. Research by Drury *et al.* (1998) found that adolescents were most likely to report good communication experiences with friends and other peers, while they experienced poor communication with non-family adults. This follows the findings by Collins and Repinski (1994), who demonstrated the importance of familiarity, equal status and shared values in teenagers' understandings of what enables good communication. Drury *et al.* (1998) also demonstrate that a greater proportion of poor communication occurs with family members rather than with their peers, and this is consistent with research that highlights family conflict in adolescence. It is during this time that family relations become strained, as the adolescent no longer sees parents as figures of authority. However, parents and other adults are continually striving to maintain their authority; consequently conflict arises (Steinberg, 1990; Bosma *et al.*, 1996). At the same time, the adolescents themselves are in the process of forming their own values which they see as being more likely to be shared within their own peer relationships than with adults (Drury *et al.*, 1998). Drury *et al.*'s (1998) study found that adolescents described particularly poor communication experiences with only one subgroup – the police. It appears that they perceive an imbalance of power in the favour of authority figures.

The above points need to be borne in mind when communicating with adolescents. Healthcare professionals must try to approach adolescents as equals. It is not necessary to know the latest vocabulary, speech patterns or text language, but it is important to respect and to listen to them. If adolescents perceive that they are being communicated with and treated fairly, they will often respond positively.

## COMMUNICATING WITH FAMILIES

Communicating with families of children is no different from communicating with children. The language/vocabulary may be different, but the underpinning strategies of communication remain the same. These include honesty and genuineness, respect, warmth, empathy and clarity (Riley, 2004). However, problems can occur when families put themselves between the children and the people caring for them. There are often good reasons for this, for example parents feel responsible for their child and expect the healthcare professionals to rely on them for information about their child's well-being (Tates *et al.*, 2002). Remember that the parents may be trying to protect the child, or they could be trying to prevent the child from communicating something distressing.

Often families will come into contact with healthcare professionals when they are feeling extremely vulnerable. This may sometimes lead to breakdowns in communication as families may not have really been listening to what they have been told, while the professionals may feel that the families may not wish, or even not be able, to make important decisions. This can lead to professionals making decisions about children rather than including their parents.

The healthcare professional needs to be aware of the vulnerability of families, and seek to communicate with them at a level that they can understand and that they can take in at any one moment. This becomes a matter of choosing the correct words (it is easy to develop a jargon that parents may not understand), the right environment and tone of voice, gestures and posture. Families need to feel that they are working with the healthcare professionals.

A study by Cuttini *et al.* (1999) on parental visiting, communication and participation in ethical dilemmas regarding sick neonates found that there was a lot of difference throughout Europe regarding parental decisions. When they looked at British neonatal units, they found that in 89% of them parents were given the opportunity to take part in decisions, even though paediatricians 'often claim to themselves the role of child advocate' (p. F88).

It is always important to remember that, although the healthcare professional may have expert knowledge, the family knows the child. They know how the child will react in different circumstances, how they behave when in pain and what they enjoy doing (this can be used as distraction therapy). Families and children often have their own personal ways of communicating, and, if he or she is sensitive enough, the healthcare professional will be able to work effectively with all concerned.

---

**Activity**
*You have seen Gemma, a 6-year-old girl, swearing at her mother and refusing to do what she is asked. Obviously, communications between the girl and her mother have broken down. What can you do to help remedy the situation?*

---

You may have thought about:

- taking Gemma away from her mother into a safe environment;
- using other communication methods – language, play, gestures, drawing – to try and find out what the problem is from Gemma's perspective;
- giving Gemma the freedom to express herself, without fear of any consequences;

- really listening to Gemma;
- giving Gemma time to settle;
- finding a private space to talk to Gemma's mother;
- being supportive, but non-committal, and discussing with the mother what the problem is, as she perceives it;
- discussing with her mother Gemma's perspective of the problem, and listening to her account;
- giving Gemma's mother time and space in order for her to consider what has happened;
- taking some time out yourself to consider what has happened and how you could possibly resolve it;
- after some time has elapsed, meeting with Gemma and her mother in a quiet, comfortable and private area;
- using appropriate methods of communication to allow Gemma and her mother to resolve the problem in a quiet and conciliatory way.

## CONCLUSION

Communication is often something that is taken for granted. However, it is an extremely complicated process. To communicate, at least two people have to be involved – the communicator and the person for whom the communication is intended. Although language is the most sophisticated and effective method of communication, other means need to be considered. This is particularly important when working with children who have developing needs and desires that they need to communicate. This chapter has identified two major means of communication, other than the spoken language, namely play and drawings. However, there are other ways in which people can express themselves. Mention has been made of gestures, expressions, posture, tone of voice, spatial relationships and touch. However, the overriding principle for the healthcare professional is to listen and interpret what has been said, ensuring that the communicator knows that they have been heard. It is only through doing this that the child's and their family's perspective can be understood and their needs met.

## REFERENCES

Allen RE (ed) (1993) *The Concise Oxford Dictionary of Current English* (8th edn). Oxford: Oxford University Press.

Bosma HA, Jackson SE, Zijsling DH *et al.* (1996) Who has the final say? Decisions on adolescent behaviour within the family. *Journal of Adolescence* 19, 227–291.

Buckley R (2003) *Children's Communication Skills: From birth to five years.* London: Routledge.

Camaioni L, Aureli T, Bellagamba F and Fogel A (2003) A longitudinal examination of the transition to symbolic communication in the second year of life. *Infant and Child Development* 12, 1–26.

Chambers AM (1993) Play as therapy for the hospitalized child. *Journal of Clinical Nursing* 2, 349–354.

Chambers W & R LTD (1998) *The Chambers Dictionary.* Edinburgh: Chambers Harrap Publishers Ltd.

Collins WA and Repinski DJ (1994) Relationships during adolescence: Continuity and change in interpersonal perspective. In Montemayer R, Adams GR and Gullotta TP (eds) *Personal Relationships During Adolescence.* Thousand Oaks, CA: SAGE.

Cooper J, Moodley M and Reynell J (1978) *Helping Language Development.* London: Edward Arnold.

Cuttini M, Rebagliato M, Bortoli P *et al.* (1999) Parental visiting, communication, and participation in ethical decisions: A comparison of neonatal unit policies in Europe. *Archives of Diseases in Childhood Fetal and Neonatal Edition* 81, F84–F91.

Department for Education and Skills (DfES) (2005) *Common Core of Skills and Knowledge for the Children's Workforce.* Nottingham: DfES.

DiLeo J (1970) *Young Children and their Drawings.* New York: Brunner/Mazel.

DiLeo J (1983) *Interpreting Children's Drawings.* New York: Brunner/Mazel.

Drury J, Catan L, Dennison C and Brody R (1998) Exploring teenagers accounts of bad communication: A new basis for intervention. *Journal of Adolescence* 21, 177–196.

Garvey C (1977) *Play* (2nd edn). London: Fontana Press.

Goldschmied E and Selleck D (1996) *Communication Between Babies in Their First Year.* London: National Children's Bureau.

Golinkoff RM and Hirsh-Pasek K (1999) *How Babies Talk: The magic and mystery of language in the first three years of life.* New York: Plume.

Hetherington EM and Parke RD (1986) *Child Psychology: A contemporary viewpoint.* New York: McGraw-Hill.

Hulse WC (1952) Childhood conflict expressed through family drawings. *Journal of Projective Techniques* 16, 66–79.

Jarvis J and Lamb S (2001) Interaction and the development of communication in the under twos: Issues for practitioners working with young children in groups. *Early Years* 21(2), 129–138.

Johnson BH (1990) Children's drawings as a projective technique. *Pediatric Nursing* 16(1), 11–17.

Kelley SJ (1985) Drawings: Critical communication for sexually abused children. *Pediatric Nursing* 11, 421–426.

Lindqvist G (2001) When small children play: How adults dramatise and children create meaning. *Early Years* 21(1), 7–14.

Linesch D (2002) Art therapy students collect children's drawings: parallel responses to September 11. *The Arts in Psychotherapy* 29, 155–157.

Oster GD, Gould P (1987) *Using Drawings in Assessment and Therapy: A guide for mental health professionals.* New York: Brunner/Mazel.

Paterson T (2005) School art from Nazi era shows children's view of Third Reich. *The Independent.* Saturday 22 October, p. 27.

Paul R (1995) *Language Disorders from Infancy through Adolescence: Assessment and intervention.* New York: Elsevier.

Pease MD, Gleason BJ and Pan AB (1989) Gaining meaning: Semantic development. In Gleason BJ (ed) *The Development of Language* (2nd edn). Columbus: Merrill Publishing.

Reynolds K (1997) *What is the Transmission Model of Interpersonal Communication and What is Wrong with it?* <file://K:\Communication\Transmission%20Model%20of%20Communication.htm> (accessed 22 August 2005).

Riley JB (2004) *Communication in Nursing* (5th edn). St Louis: Mosby.

Steinberg L (1990) Autonomy, conflict and harmony in the family relationship. In Feldman SS and Elliott GR (eds) *At the Threshold: The developing adolescence.* Cambridge, MA: Harvard University Press.

Shannon CE and Weaver W (1949) *The Mathematical Theory of Communication.* Urbana, IL: University of Illinois Press.

Tager-Flusberg H (1989) Putting words together: morphology and syntax in the pre-school years. In: Gleason JB (ed) *The Development of Language* (2nd edn). Columbus: Merrill Publishing.

Tates K, Meeuwesen L, Elbers E and Bensing J (2002) I've come for his throat: Roles and identities in doctor–parent–child communication. *Child: Care, Health & Development* 28(1), 109–116.

Thomas GV and Silk AMJ (1990) *An Introduction to the Psychology of Children's Drawings.* Hemel Hempstead: Harvester/Wheatsheaf.

Umek LM and Musek PL (2001) Symbolic play: Opportunities for cognitive and language development in preschool settings. *Early Years* 21(1), 55–64.

Veltman MWM and Browne KD (2001) Identifying childhood abuse through favorite kind of day and kinetic family drawings. *The Arts in Psychotherapy* 28, 251–259.

Vickers PS (1999) *Severe Combined Immunodeficiency Syndrome: A pediatric emergency and a chronic disease?* PhD Thesis.

Walker SC (1998) Stories of two children: Making sense of children's therapeutic work. *The Arts in Psychotherapy* 25(4), 263–275.

# 4 Working as a Member of the Child Health Team

## L. WHITING AND I. PEATE

## INTRODUCTION

Bekaert (2005) suggests that the contribution of all professionals is essential in order to safeguard the needs of children. Caring for children and their families is complex, and there is a need to liaise and communicate with a range of health and social-care professionals from various statutory and voluntary agencies. This chapter will consider the roles of key personnel and how they interface with each other to facilitate the provision of high-quality care. The principles of effective communication discussed in Chapter 3 will be developed further, and the skills required to participate effectively as a member of the multidisciplinary team will be explored. However, first of all, an overview of the National Health Service (NHS) will be provided to facilitate an understanding of this large and diverse organisation that employs the largest team of healthcare professionals in the UK.

## THE ORGANISATION OF HEALTH CARE IN THE UK: THE NHS

The majority of health care in the UK is delivered by the NHS. It was established in 1948 and is a large and complex organisation that is now Europe's largest single employer. It has undergone numerous reforms and reorganisations over the years.

It is estimated that there are over 1 166 000 people employed in the NHS in England. Approximately two-thirds of those contribute to direct care – the delivery of health care – these people include registered nurses (RNs) and health care assistants (HCAs) (Department of Health (DH), 2005) (Table 4.1).

The *NHS Plan* (DH, 2000) resulted in the biggest changes in the NHS since its inception. It outlined a 10-year strategy of investment in relation to the reform of NHS provision for patients. In addition, devolution had an impor-

*Caring for Children and Families.* Edited by I. Peate and L. Whiting
© 2006 John Wiley & Sons Ltd

**Table 4.1** Estimations related to the numbers of healthcare staff employed by the NHS (Source: Geldman, 2002)

| Professional Group | Approximations |
|---|---|
| Administrative and estates staff | 224 000 |
| Scientific, therapeutic and technical employees | 115 000 |
| Medical and dental workforce | 74 000 |
| Consultants | 26 000 |
| General practitioners (GPs) | 30 600 |

tant impact on how healthcare services function in the four countries of the UK. There are significant differences in the operation of the NHS; the following four figures (4.1, 4.2, 4.3 and 4.4) outline the structure of the NHS in England, Wales, Scotland and Northern Ireland.

## THE STRUCTURE OF THE NHS IN ENGLAND

This section will consider in further detail the structure of the NHS in England, the largest healthcare provider in the UK.

### The Department of Health

The DH is responsible for leading the NHS in social care as well as improving standards of public health. The Secretary of State works with five other Ministers for Health and a range of other executive figures, for example the NHS Chief Executive. The Secretary of State is accountable to Parliament for the function of the NHS. Key responsibilities of the DH are highlighted below:

- setting overall direction
- ensuring that national standards are set
- securing resources
- deciding on major investments
- improving choice for patients and service users.

### Strategic Health Authorities

There are 28 Strategic Health Authorities (SHAs); these were established in 2002. SHAs have the same boundaries as local authorities (which are responsible for the provision of social services) and provide health care for approximately 1.5 million people, from birth to old age.

SHAs manage local NHS services and are closely linked to the DH. Each SHA has produced its own local delivery plan based on national priorities and the aims of each Primary Care Trust (PCT).

**ENGLAND**

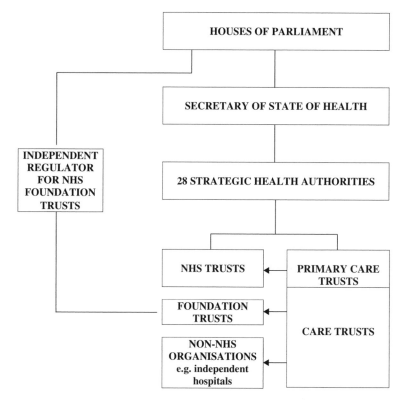

**Figure 4.1** The structure of the NHS in England, April 2004 *(source: Association of Clinical Pathologists (ACP), 2004).*

SHAs have four key roles:

1. to develop coherent strategies associated with the improvement of the local health service;
2. to ensure high-quality performance of the local health service and its organisations, working towards improved performance;
3. to build capacity into the local health service to ensure wide provision of services;
4. to make certain that priorities that have been agreed upon, on a national level, are integrated into local health plans.

### Primary Care Trusts

Of the overall NHS budget 75% is directed towards PCTs. There are just over 300 PCTs, each with a population of approximately 150 000 to 300 000 people.

WALES

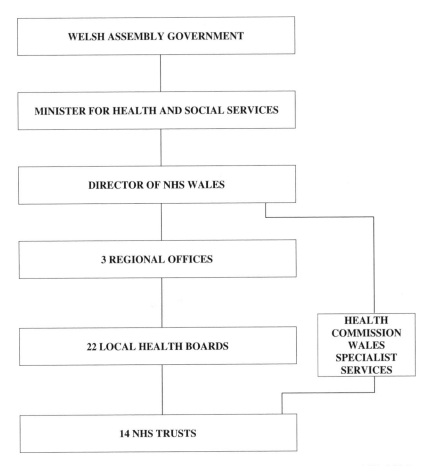

**Figure 4.2** The structure of the NHS in Wales, April 2004 *(source: ACP, 2004).*

PCTs are the cornerstone of the NHS (ACP, 2004). Broadly, they have three key roles:

1. to plan and secure health services for the local populations; this will include determining which health services the local population needs and ensuring that those services are provided;
2. to improve the health of their local population;
3. to integrate health care and social care at a local level.

### Care Trusts

Care Trusts are organisations that work in both health and social care. They can carry out a range of services for example:

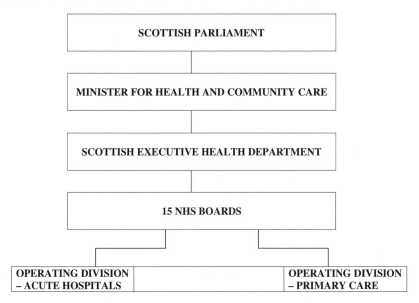

**Figure 4.3** The structure of the NHS in Scotland, April 2004 *(source: ACP, 2004)*

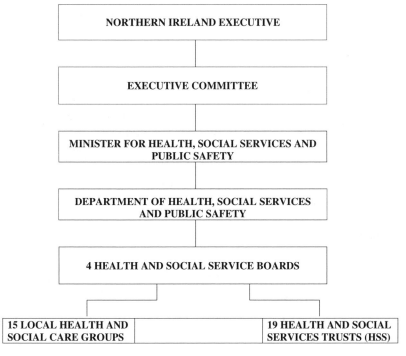

**Figure 4.4** The structure of the NHS in Northern Ireland, April 2004 *(source: ACP, 2004).*

- social care
- mental health services
- primary care services.

Care Trusts are set up when the NHS and Local Authorities agree to work closely together, often this is carried out when a closer relationship is required between health care and social care.

### NHS Trusts

NHS Trusts run the majority of hospitals. They work closely with the PCTs and are accountable to the SHAs as opposed to being directly accountable to the DH.

### Foundation Trusts

These Trusts have only been established since 2004. They are free-standing organisations with greater independence within the NHS (DH, 2002). Foundation trusts are non-profit-making organisations and are owned by their members, who are local people, employees and other key stakeholders. Foundation Trusts are accountable through various arrangements, that is through the Independent Regulator; the Commission for Health Care Audit and Inspection and service level agreements with the PCTs.

### Special Health Authorities

In addition to the above, a number of Special Health Authorities (SpHAs) have been established to provide the NHS with a nationwide service. The SpHAs are independent entities, but they are subjected to ministerial direction like other NHS bodies. SpHAs include the:

- National Institute for Health and Clinical Excellence (NICE)
- National Clinical Assessment Authority
- National Patient Safety Agency
- National Blood Transfusion Authority.

## PRIMARY, SECONDARY AND TERTIARY HEALTHCARE SERVICES

There are various aspects of care offered by the NHS that are often referred to as:

- acute care
- chronic care.

Care also occurs within the following healthcare settings:

- primary
- secondary
- tertiary.

## Acute care

Children who have acute care problems have a rapid onset of disease that does not usually last a long time, often they respond quickly to treatment and a full recovery is expected; prolonged care is not normally required. Children experiencing acute problems may receive care in the home (with the support of the GP, the community children's nurse or the health visitor), on a hospital ward or in an accident and emergency department. The following are some examples of acute problems in childhood:

- appendicitis
- otitis media
- febrile convulsions.

Although manifestations of these acute problems are short and intense, the child may have clinical symptoms for approximately 30 days. It is important to remember that acute conditions are usually reversible (Neander and Holmes, 2004).

## Chronic care or long-term care

Children who receive long-term care generally have an illness that is characterised by a gradual, insidious onset that may cause a disruption in functional ability. Chronic conditions are usually irreversible and lifelong changes are needed to help the child and family cope (Neander and Holmes, 2004). Examples of chronic childhood problems include:

- sickle-cell disease
- Duchenne's muscular dystrophy
- cerebral palsy
- cystic fibrosis.

## Primary care services

Often people think that most care takes place within the hospital setting, when in actual fact over 95 % of care is delivered in the primary care sector. Primary care is care that is delivered outside hospitals by a range of practitioners, for example:

- teams of nurses (e.g. community children's nurses, school nurses, children's clinical nurse specialists, children's nurse consultants)

- groups of doctors (e.g. GPs, community children's consultants)
- midwives
- health visitors
- dentists
- pharmacists
- optometrists
- child psychologists
- occupational therapists
- physiotherapists
- speech therapists.

For a great many children and their families, the professional health care they need will be carried out in the community setting. The DH aims to provide a 'one-stop shop service' for all children and families needing primary care.

However, in certain circumstances, the care provided by the primary care sector may not be appropriate, or able, to meet the needs of the child and family. As a result, referral to other services is required – those services are offered by the secondary care sector.

### Secondary care services

Secondary care provision occurs mainly through the acute hospital setting where the child and family should be cared for by children's nurses and paediatricians. The nursing and medical staff who work in this area have more readily available access to specialist and elaborate diagnostic aids and facilities, for example:

- X-ray department
- magnetic resonance imaging (MRI)
- computer axial tomography (CAT) scans
- operating theatres
- special care baby units (SCBU)
- microbiological laboratories.

Those who provide care in the primary care setting, for example the community children's nurse and GP may be seen as the gatekeeper to care provision in the secondary care sector, as they may make the necessary referrals. For the child and family, the transition from primary care to secondary care should be a seamless move. The distinction between the two is becoming blurred since a child may visit hospital for just a few hours before having follow-up care in the community.

### Tertiary care services

In some larger hospitals, there may be an opportunity to provide the child with tertiary care. Tertiary care is provided by children's nurses and paediatricians with specialist expertise, equipment and facilities for caring for children and their families with complex healthcare needs, for example:

- paediatric intensive care units (PICU)
- neonatal units
- burns units
- oncology centres.

The staff working in these areas will usually have undertaken additional courses to enable them to further develop their skills and knowledge – tertiary care may provide an avenue for career development. It is important to remember that the majority of children and their families will receive their care and have their needs met in the primary care setting. Only a few will require the services of those who work in the secondary care sector, and even fewer will need to access services provided in tertiary care.

Figure 4.5 provides a diagrammatic representation of primary, secondary and tertiary care services using the Children's Cardiac Liaison Nursing Service to illustrate the point.

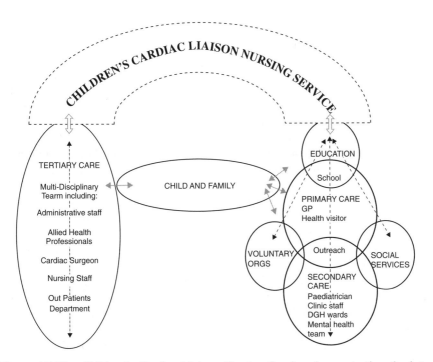

**Figure 4.5** The Children's Cardiac Liaison Nursing Service, demonstrating the integration of primary, secondary and tertiary services. *(Reproduced with the kind permission of Margaret Jiggins, Royal Brompton and Harefield NHS Trust.)*

## COMMUNICATING WITH HEALTHCARE PROFESSIONALS

In order to communicate effectively with other healthcare professionals, it is important to know who these people are. There are many people that the child and family will come into contact with. If you act as the child's advocate, it is important to understand not only your own role but also that of others providing healthcare delivery.

The Nursing and Midwifery Council (NMC) (2004) requires that all RNs, midwives and specialist community public health nurses work in collaboration with the patient and other healthcare professionals in order to enhance and promote high-quality care. Good-quality and effective communication in healthcare teams has the potential to contribute to the introduction of new and improved ways of delivering patient care.

*The National Service Framework for Children, Young People and Maternity Services* (DH and DfES, 2004) suggests that one of the markers of good practice is that there is continuity between care delivered in the various health settings. The sharing of relevant information between healthcare professionals must be supported by systems that ensure that this is done in a suitable manner. Children and their families come into contact with the NHS via a range of channels at different times; because of this, there is a possibility that care may become disjointed (DH and DfES, 2004). The sharing of relevant information with the appropriate healthcare professional is therefore vital if this is to be avoided.

Patient Advice and Liaison Services (PALS) have been initiated in all NHS Trusts and PCTs; the child and family may come into contact with this service. The creation of PALS was as a result of the *NHS Plan* (DH, 2000) and was aimed at enabling patients, and the public, to access information and raise concerns with their Trust – the service provides on-the-spot help. While the work of PALS is growing, the adequacy of existing resources in relation to children, young people and parents needs to be given further deliberation (Heaton and Sloper, 2003).

The NHS is not the only agency providing health care and social care. There are many voluntary and charitable groups that offer a range of different services for children and families. For example, young people with mental health problems may benefit from the facilities offered by MIND (a leading mental health charity) that provides day-centre care and befriending schemes. Other organisations, such as the Meningitis Trust, the Down's Syndrome Association, Asthma UK and the Cystic Fibrosis Trust, all have a range of valuable services – bear this in mind when thinking about with whom you may need to communicate.

Consider the scenario below and take some time to think about whom Jeannine and her family may come into contact with after she has been admitted to hospital, and then again after she has been transferred to the hospice.

**Table 4.2** The healthcare professionals Jeannine and her family may have come into contact with

| | |
|---|---|
| • children's nurses | • medical staff (e.g. GPs, consultants and specialist registrars) |
| • school nurse | |
| • health visitor | • speech therapist |
| • community children's nurses (especially those specialising in continuing care) | • paediatric occupational therapist |
| | • paediatric social worker |
| • student nurses | • family therapist |
| • healthcare assistants | • child psychologist |
| • paediatric physiotherapists | • technicians |
| • domestic and portering staff | • dietitian |
| | • PALS officer |
| | • voluntary and charitable organisations |

**Activity**

*Jeannine is a 6-year-old girl who was born with a condition known as microcephaly. At birth, she was seriously ill and was nursed in the SCBU of a tertiary care setting for three months. When Jeannine was 2 years of age, her mother left the family and now has little contact with them. Since this time, Jeannine has been living at home with her father and her two older sisters.*

*Jeannine has a range of complex health needs, and her family realise that she has a life-limiting condition. She has required much nursing support since her birth and her father has managed to care for her with the help of a range of healthcare professionals – predominantly from primary care services. Over the last two weeks, Jeannine's condition has deteriorated and seven days ago she was admitted to her local children's unit (an acute care ward) with a diagnosis of pneumonia.*

*Her father has now agreed that she be transferred to a children's hospice for a month of respite care.*

Jeannine and her family will have come into contact with many healthcare professionals, you may have thought about those listed in Table 4.2.

## MEMBERS OF THE MULTIDISCIPLINARY TEAM

NURSING STAFF

The largest group of healthcare professionals employed by the NHS are the 397515 qualified nurses (DH, 2005). *Making a Difference* (DH, 1999) sets out the Government's strategic intentions for nursing, midwifery and health visiting; these intentions include the establishment of a nursing career framework (Figure 4.6).

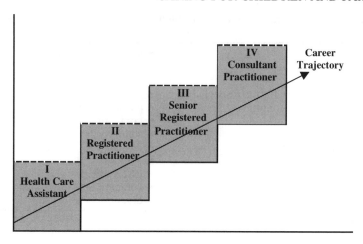

**Figure 4.6** Nursing career framework *(source: DH, 1999).*

### Chief Nursing Officer

The Chief Nursing Officer (CNO), a civil servant, is the Government's most senior nursing adviser and has the responsibility to ensure that the Government's strategy for nursing, *Making a Difference* (DH, 1999), is delivered. The CNO leads over 597 625 nurses, midwives and health visitors and other allied health professionals.

### Nurse consultant

Nurse consultants are experienced and expert practitioners; there are now a new range of these posts within children's nursing practice, within both hospital and community settings. One of the key aims of the post is to strengthen professional leadership, but there are four main areas of responsibility (DH, 1999):

- expert practice
- professional leadership and consultancy
- education and development
- practice and service development linked to research and evaluation.

Most paediatric nurse consultants spend approximately 50% of their time in clinical practice in direct contact with children and families; their remaining time may be spent undertaking research, teaching, leadership and evaluation activities.

### Ward sister/charge nurse/ward manager

Ward sisters and their male counterparts, charge nurses, are experienced practitioners who have developed extensive skills and knowledge in their chosen area, for example:

- SCBU
- child and adolescent mental health unit
- paediatric oncology
- children's nursing within a general hospital
- community practice
- PICU.

The ward sister/charge nurse has many responsibilities, including leadership, acting as a role model and facilitating staff learning.

### Staff nurse

The staff nurse has completed a minimum of three years' education, usually at a higher education institution (HEI) and may be required as he or she gains more experience to act as deputy for the ward sister/charge nurse. Usually, the staff nurse has her or his own group of children to care for within the hospital or community setting. More experienced staff nurses can become facilitators/mentors to other junior members of the team.

### Student nurse

Entry requirements to become a student nurse have been devolved to the local HEIs, which provide nurse-education programmes. All candidates apply through the UCAS (Universities and Colleges Admissions Service) for the degree pathway, or NMAS (Nursing and Midwifery Admissions Service) for the diploma pathway. In addition, the Government has made plans to widen entry into professional education for those who do not posses the 'traditional' requirements (DH, 1999). Chapter 13 discusses student nurses and possible career routes in more detail.

All nursing students undertake a programme of study that is three years full time, and graduate with an academic as well as a professional qualification (the latter providing registration with the NMC – their licence to practise). All programmes offer the opportunity to study for 50% of the time in clinical areas (including community and institutional settings) and the remaining 50% undertaking theoretical work, usually at the HEI.

### Healthcare assistants and cadet nurses

HCAs provide clinical support to healthcare professionals in many settings. They often undertake vocational qualifications as a part of their job, and in some HEIs, in an attempt to widen access to nurse-education programmes, the vocational qualification may meet the academic entry requirement to a programme of study leading to professional nursing registration.

The concept of cadet nurses has been reintroduced over the last few years, again with the key aim of encouraging a wider entry route to the more formal study of nurse education. The programmes are usually of two years' duration, leading to a vocational award and are normally joint ventures between NHS Trusts and local further education (FE) colleges.

## MEDICAL STAFF

### Chief Medical Officer

Just as the CNO is the most senior nurse adviser to the Government, the Chief Medical Officer (CMO) is the most senior doctor and is also a civil servant. There are separate CMOs for England, Scotland, Wales and Northern Ireland.

### Consultant

The consultant is a specialist in medicine who has undertaken further study. Consultant paediatricians may work in a variety of settings, including primary, secondary and tertiary care areas. It is the consultant who accepts overall responsibility for the child's care.

### General practitioner

The GP works in the community and provides family health services to a local area. He or she may work alone (single-handed practice) or with other GPs (group practice). GPs often refer children with more complex conditions to a paediatric consultant. There are some GPs who have completed a course specifically related to children.

### General practitioner registrar

General practitioner registrars (GPRs) are vocational posts that provide doctors with the skills, knowledge and competences necessary to work in a GP practice; they are doctors who are learning in the GP setting.

### Specialist registrar

The specialist registrar (SpR) (paediatrics) has replaced the former senior registrar (SR) post. The SpR has to have completed a defined college or faculty specialist education programme prior to obtaining the post. Having completed this course of study, he or she is eligible to apply for a consultant's position. Alternatively, he or she may take on more clinical responsibility and become a clinical assistant.

**Senior house officer/house officer**

Having graduated from medical school, the house officer (HO) must undertake one year's hospital experience as a requirement of the General Medical Council (GMC) prior to being able to register as a doctor. Once registered with the GMC, he or she may apply to become a senior house officer (SHO) with opportunities to experience paediatric medicine.

**Medical student**

Most medical students in the UK will graduate with bachelors' degrees in medicine and surgery (MB, MS). Each medical school sets its own entry requirements to study medicine and candidates apply through UCAS. During their course, all will study paediatrics.

Clearly, there are many other healthcare professionals whom you may meet and work with (such as physiotherapists, radiographers and social workers). However, this section of the chapter has focused on the two professions (nursing and medicine) that you will almost certainly encounter when working with children and their families. Being aware of the roles of other healthcare professionals can facilitate your ability to work as a member of the multidisciplinary team. Great emphasis has been placed on the development of integrated teams in the *NHS Plan* (DH, 2000) – everyone has a responsibility to strive towards this goal to enhance patient care.

## TEAM WORKING

Working as a member of a team is a key characteristic for all healthcare professionals. There are various teams of different sizes and structures within the healthcare setting. It is important that you work as an effective member of your team in order to support colleagues as well as the children and their families. The following section will discuss the factors that influence effective teamwork; in addition, it outlines your role and function as a team member.

Kekki (1990) for the World Health Organisation (WHO) defines 'teamwork' as coordinated action that is undertaken by two or more individuals either jointly, concurrently or sequentially. Teams have commonly agreed goals, respect and awareness of others' roles and functions. Trust, effective leadership and open, honest and sensitive communication are all key components of an effective team. Johnson (2004) states that a team is a group of people who often represent various professions and who may work together to attain and achieve certain goals and plans of action to meet the needs of the patient.

The need to work together as a team has been stressed in *The NHS Plan* (DH, 2000) and *Shifting the Balance of Power* (DH, 2001a). A growing body of evidence suggests that team working can have a significant impact not only on the quality of care but also on the efficient use of resources and staff satisfaction (DH, 2001b). The best and most cost-effective outcomes for children and families will be achieved when professionals work together in order to ensure the child and family are at the centre of care (Borrill et al., 2000).

With the many advances in healthcare technology, new ways of working and managing care are continually emerging. Influences such as the use of telemedicine and the computerisation of patient records have had a positive impact on patient care (Smith, 2004). As organisations such as the NHS grow in size and become even more complex, there is a need for teams of people to work in a more coordinated way to achieve the objectives that have been set (Borrill et al., 2000).

Team working is seen as an essential pre-requisite to modern health care. Wakley et al. (2003) suggest that in order to work competently the team should:

- share information;
- ask others for their views and share own views;
- listen to others' ideas and challenges constructively;
- build on the ideas of others;
- support the team's decisions and put team needs above personal interests;
- seek resolution of differences between team members;
- meet commitments given to the team;
- alert the team when it is deviating from its task.

A large research study by Borrill et al. (2000) was undertaken to investigate the effectiveness of healthcare teams in the NHS. Effective teams, according to Borrill et al. (2000), will have:

- clear objectives;
- higher levels of team members participating in decision-making;
- a strong commitment to quality;
- support for innovation.

## PHASES IN TEAM DEVELOPMENT

Before a team can become fully functional, it must go through several 'influential' stages. Four key stages have been identified by Tuckman as far back as 1965 (Tuckman, 1965); these are the phases that a team needs to go through to become fully established and effective (see Table 4.3).

Figure 4.7 provides a diagrammatic representation of the four stages.

Later, Tuckman added a fifth dimension to his model – the adjourning stage (Tuckman and Jensen, 1975). This is associated with the break-up of the group, occurring when the task has been successfully completed. For example, when the child has been discharged from hospital, the purpose has been fulfilled and the team members can move on to new things.

**Table 4.3** Phases associated with group development
*(Source: Adapted from Tuckman, 1965)*

**Forming stage**
This first stage is characterised by uncertainty about purpose and structure. There is much dependence on the leader for guidance and support. The leader tends to direct the group. Team members start to feel their way, and it is only when they begin to think of themselves as a team that they move on to the second stage.

**Storming stage**
Group conflict may occur at this stage, with each group experiencing and displaying professional rivalry. There tends to be some vying for position and decision-making is difficult. An overwhelming issue of who has control and who holds the power becomes central. Cliques and factions may form and there can be power struggles. The leader tends to take on the role of coach.

**Norming stage**
The third stage sees unity emerging as a result of conflict. Group identity now becomes apparent along with group values replacing individualism. Roles and responsibilities emerge. The leader is now seen as a facilitator and enabler.

**Performing stage**
The group is much more solid in this, the final stage, and each team member knows her/his place. The team is more strategically aware during the performing stage; the team knows clearly why and what it is doing. The key aim is to achieve as a group, by taking on group tasks. Group dynamics, once an important part of the development process, are now less important. The leader delegates and oversees.

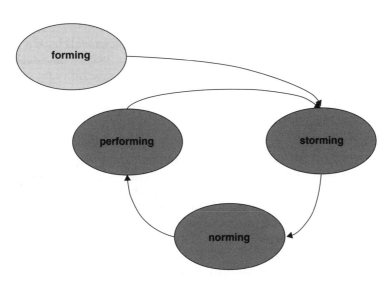

**Figure 4.7** The forming, storming, norming and performing model *(source: Tuckman, 1965).*

The developmental model above can aid understanding of how small groups may come together as a multidisciplinary team in order to meet aims and objectives. The model, despite being more than 40 years old, reflects the fact that small groups do appear to follow a rather predictable course.

## TEAM WORKING IN CLINICAL PRACTICE

### Negotiation skills

Being able to negotiate successfully is a skill you will need to develop; it is a personal skill and is necessary to resolve conflict or to come to common agreement about goals and aims that have been planned. This is particularly relevant when working with children and families as this provides a united strategy and can limit confusion.

Negotiation can be both formal and informal (Martin, 1998). You have already developed a range of informal negotiation skills – think about when you and your friends decide to go out for a meal; you negotiate where to meet and at what time. Formal negotiation occurs when there are differences that need to be resolved and agreements made. For example, there may be a difference of opinion about a particular feeding method for a child with cerebral palsy who requires continuing care. This formal approach should allow all parties to have their opinions and obligations formally recorded.

According to Makinson (2000), reaching agreement through negotiation is a feature of everyday working life. He suggests that using tactics to negotiate effectively can help with the handling of disagreements and conflict – certainly something that is important when working as a team member. There may be disagreement and conflict within the team and also between the team, the child and the family. Do remember that all healthcare professionals have a responsibility to always act in the child's best interests (DH, 1989) – this in itself can provoke conflict if parents, children or professionals have different opinions.

### Uni- and multidisciplinary team models

Unidisciplinary teamwork is described by Lowe and O'Hara (2000) as a model of service provision where professionals from the same discipline are grouped together into departments and are accountable for matters from that discipline. This can result in care being profession-led. In this way, the focus of care is often based on the delivery of a specialist service across a range of client groups. Such an approach may call into question issues surrounding efficacy and efficiency of care provision. Øvretveit et al. (1997) point out that when different professions fail to work together duplication, mistakes and delays can occur.

The unidisciplinary team model has limitations and there are alternative working strategies. One other approach is to embrace the multidisciplinary team model. This system of care delivery has the potential to improve care provision and reduce the duplication often associated with the unidisciplinary approach (Wheelan and Hochberger, 1996), for example parents being asked the same questions over and over again by different healthcare professionals (Carter, 2004).

The multidisciplinary team approach, according to Hands and Wilson (1997), can reduce the variation often seen in clinical practice by bringing together the skills of the team with child- and family-focused outcomes. This approach also coordinates the expertise of a range of healthcare professionals, thereby pooling resources and making more effective and efficient use of both human and physical resources. However, it must be remembered that the formation of multidisciplinary teams will not be the answer to all of the problems and challenges you may face when working with the child and family; the team must still strive to work effectively.

In order to work as an effective team member you need to:

- have a positive attitude towards the child and her or his family and listen to their wishes and needs;
- make sure that the child, family and other colleagues understand the roles and responsibilities of team members;
- be aware of what the child and family think about the quality of services offered;
- have a clear understanding of professional values, standards and purpose;
- be willing to learn and accept learning as a lifelong process;
- be committed to providing good-quality effective care;
- respect the skills and contributions of colleagues, children and families;
- be open and honest about professional performance;
- try to challenge other team members when there is a belief that a decision could harm a child.

There may be occasions when you are concerned that the decision or action of others is not in the best interests of the child or their family. If this occurs, try to use your negotiation skills; if you are still unhappy about the situation, refer the matter to someone who can take further action, for example a senior nurse manager.

It is important to understand the role of other members of the team and to value the purpose of multidisciplinary working. It is also crucial to understand your own role, how you interact with others in the team and the contribution you make to the care of the child and family. Northcott (2003) recognises that there may be professional rivalry occurring in the team. This conflict can be the cause of poor performance among different members. The team may need to be reminded that it is the collective efforts of everyone which are important and that, while they will and do occur, differences should be acknowledged and respected. Conflict that occurs must be recognised and managed by the team – it can be useful to plan a specific meeting to facilitate the solving of problems.

There may be various opportunities where the healthcare team meets in order to discuss care issues, for example:

- case conferences to review a child's progress, care, management and organisation of discharge arrangements;
- ward rounds to discuss progress, to review care provision and to provide direction;
- legal or statutory attendance at a court hearing to provide evidence;
- GP practice meetings to consider overall strategies for children and families;
- school meetings to discuss one particular child, a group of children or to discuss the implementation of a policy.

No matter where any of these meetings take place, the overriding principle is to promote and ensure confidentiality and to act in the child's best interests (DH, 1989). Section 5.1 of the NMC code of professional conduct, standards for conduct, performance and ethics (NMC, 2004) states that any information obtained about patients and clients must be treated as confidential and used only for the purpose for which it was given.

Consider the scenario in the activity below and take some time to think who in the multidisciplinary team may be involved in Sanjay's care and the roles that each member may play.

---

**Activity**

*Sanjay is 12 years old and was playing football at school when he hurt his little finger of his left hand. His teacher referred him to the school nurse – she examined the injury (the affected area was slightly swollen and sore) and then contacted Sanjay's mother to request that she took him home. Later that evening, Sanjay's finger developed extensive swelling and his parents took him to the paediatric assessment unit (PAU) at his local hospital. While at the PAU, Sanjay underwent a full assessment, including an X-ray, and was diagnosed with a fracture of the proximal phalanx of the finger. His finger was strapped to the adjacent finger and Sanjay was given an appointment to attend fracture clinic the next day.*

---

Although Sanjay sustained a relatively minor injury, and one which should not present any long-term problems, it is interesting to consider how many members of the multidisciplinary team could have been involved in his care – this further demonstrates the need for clear and accurate communication strategies. You may have identified the following people.

- **The teacher:** He or she made the referral to the school nurse, a first and important step. Failure of prompt action on the teacher's part could have altered the course and outcome of Sanjay's injury.
- **School nurse:** A pivotal role was played by the school nurse, who was able to assess the injury, provide immediate first aid, comfort and reassure Sanjay, contact his parents and provide relevant health advice.

- **The student nurse:** The student nurse can provide support to Sanjay and his family practically and emotionally. The student nurse is also ideally placed to provide feedback through observation to the registered nurse and other healthcare workers with regards to Sanjay's health status.
- **Parents:** Sanjay's family were crucial to his care. It is his parents who monitored his condition at home and decided if further medical intervention was required. In addition, they may have acted as an advocate for Sanjay while he was in the PAU, particularly as they would have been able to inform staff about the physical changes to the injury and how Sanjay had been emotionally affected by it. Most importantly, it is Sanjay's parents who would have been best placed to comfort him. Parents have an enormous contribution to make to the overall physical, social and psychological health of their children – this should be nurtured and never underestimated. This stance is reinforced in Section 4.1 of NMC (2004), which states that the family, along with the multidisciplinary team, should be included in the provision of care.
- **PAU:**
  - Children's nurse: Sanjay will have been cared for by a children's nurse in the PAU. The nurse will have had the skills required to conduct a full assessment of Sanjay and his health needs. In addition, the nurse will have administered prescribed drugs (e.g. for the relief of pain) and will have provided the care and management required for Sanjay's injury. A significant aspect of the role may have been reassuring the family and providing information and advice about the fracture.
  - Medical staff: Sanjay will have been examined by at least one doctor (possibly more). This person will have been an experienced paediatric accident and emergency practitioner and will have decided, in negotiation with the children's nurse, the most appropriate treatment for Sanjay's finger. This doctor will also have prescribed any medication.
  - Radiographer: Sanjay's X-ray will have been carried out by a qualified radiographer, who would have been able to provide some advice in relation to the radiographic findings.
  - HCA: Sanjay's care may have been supported by an HCA, who may have accompanied Sanjay to X-ray, provided psychological reassurance and given him a game, comic or book to keep him amused while waiting for his X-ray. In addition, the HCA may have assisted the children's nurse with care and management activities.
  - Receptionist: It is important that this person had a friendly and approachable manner so that Sanjay and his parents did not feel intimidated by the strange environment – this will have assisted in the reduction of anxiety levels. The receptionist should have explained where the family should go and what facilities were available and may have arranged the fracture-clinic appointment.
- **Fracture clinic:** While in the fracture clinic, there will have been another team of staff for the family to meet, these include:

○ receptionist
○ nurse
○ orthopaedic registrar.

One of the main purposes of team working is to provide high-quality care for the child and their family. Building a successful partnership with other members of the healthcare team does take time and effort, but developing your own interpersonal skills will enhance your confidence as well as your ability to communicate effectively with all professionals, children and families.

Traditional roles and job boundaries associated with nurses and doctors are changing, for example nurses now have greater prescribing powers, thus freeing doctors' time for other activities. The role and function of all healthcare professionals is in a constant state of flux, being aware and respecting this may help you to function more effectively as a team member.

## CONCLUSION

The overriding principle when working as a member of the healthcare team is to become involved in the provision of a service that sets the child and their family at the centre. There can be no doubt that team working is a key component of quality care (Modernisation Agency, 2003); therefore, we all have a responsibility to strive to become good team players.

## REFERENCES

Association of Clinical Pathologists (ACP) (2004) *The ACP Guide to the Structure of the NHS in the United Kingdom*. East Sussex: ACP.

Bekaert S (2005) *Adolescents and Sex: The handbook for professionals working with young people*. Oxford: Radcliffe Publishing.

Borrill CS, Carletta J, Carter AJ, Dawson JF, Garrod S, Rees A *et al.* (2000) *The Effectiveness of Health Care Teams in the National Health Service*. Birmingham: Aston University.

Carter B (2004) Editorial: If I have to say it one more time, I swear I'm gonna kill someone. *Journal of Child Health Care* 8(3), 178–179.

Department of Health (DH) (1989) *The Children Act*. London: HMSO.

Department of Health (DH) (1999) *Making a Difference: Strengthening the nursing, midwifery and health visiting contribution to health and health care*. London: DH.

Department of Health (DH) (2000) *The NHS Plan a Plan for Investment: A plan for reform*. London: DH.

Department of Health (DH) (2001a) *Shifting the Balance of Power Within the NHS: Securing delivery*. London: DH.

Department of Health (DH) (2001b) *The Effectiveness of Health Care Teams in the National Health Service*. London: DH.

Department of Health (DH) (2002) *A Guide to NHS Foundation Trusts*. London: DH.

Department of Health (DH) (2005) *Staff in the NHS 2004*. London: DH.

Department of Health and Department for Education and Skills (DH/DfES) (2004) *National Service Framework for Children, Young People and Maternity Services: Children and young people who are ill*. London: DH/DfES.

Geldman A (2002) How many people does the NHS employ? The *Guardian* 26 June.

Hands D and Wilson J (1997) Integrated care management. *Health Services Journal* 107(supplement), 4–5.

Heaton J and Sloper P (2003) *Access to and Use of Patient Advice and Liaison Services (PALS) by Children, Young People and Parents: A national survey*. Social Policy Research Unit, University of York.

Johnson L (2004) *Social Work Practice* (8th edn). Boston: Allyn and Bacon.

Kekki P (1990) *Teamwork in Primary Health Care*. Geneva: World Health Organisation.

Lowe F and O'Hara S (2000) Multi-disciplinary team working in practice: managing the transition. *Journal of Interprofessional Care* 14(3), 271–279.

Makinson G (2000) Developing your negotiation skills. *Nursing and Residential Care* 4(6), 283–285.

Martin J (1998) *Organizational Behaviour*. London: Thompson Business Press.

Modernisation Agency (2003) *Team Working for Improvement: Planning for spread and sustainability*. London: Modernisation Agency.

Neander W and Holmes SB (2004) Health maintenance, health promotion, and wellness. In: Daniels R (ed) *Nursing Fundamentals: Caring and clinical decision making*, Chapter 32, pp 847–937. New York: Thompson.

Northcott N (2003) Working within a health care team. In: Hinchliff S, Norman S and Schober J (eds) *Nursing Practice and Health Care* (4th edn), Chapter 16, pp 371–389. London: Arnold.

Nursing and Midwifery Council (NMC) (2004) *The NMC Code of Professional Conduct: Standards for conduct, performance and ethics*. London: NMC.

Øvretveit J, Mathias P and Thompson T (1997) *Interprofessional Working for Health and Social Care*. London: Macmillian Press.

Smith A (2004) New ways of working. In: Chilton S, Melling K, Drew D and Clarridge A (eds) *Nursing in the Community: An essential guide to practice*, Chapter 2, pp 7–15. London: Arnold.

Tuckman BW (1965) Development sequencing in small groups. *Psychological Bulletin* 63, 384–399.

Tuckman BW and Jensen MC (1975) Stages of small group development revisited. *Group and Organisational Studies* 2, 419–427.

Wakley G, Cunnion M and Chambers R (2003) *Improving Sexual Health Advice*. Oxford: Radcliffe.

Wheelan SA and Hochberger JM (1996) Assessing the functional level of rehabilitation teams and facilitating team development. *Rehabilitation Nursing* 21, 75–80.

# 5 Health Promotion: A Child-centred Approach

**S. MILLER**

## INTRODUCTION

This chapter will provide an introduction to child health promotion. First of all, health and some of the factors that may impact upon a child's health will be considered; this will be followed by a discussion of the concept of health promotion. The challenges in identifying and meeting the health-promotion needs of children will be demonstrated through the use of three child-focused activities. Ethical issues will be raised, particularly in relation to young children who are unable to make their needs and wishes known. Finally, some of the difficulties associated with the evaluation of health promotion will be explored.

## WHY IS CHILD HEALTH IMPORTANT?

Before discussing child health and child health promotion, it would be helpful to consider why the health of children is so important. Children living in the UK are healthier than ever before and death during childhood is now rare. While this is good, it is evident that much preventable adult ill health has its roots in childhood (DH and DfES, 2004). This may be due to the environment in which the person was raised, or it could be caused by habits adopted in younger years, such as smoking. The Government has stated:

> improving the health and welfare of parents and their children is the surest way to a healthier nation. (DH and DfES, 2004, p. 8)

No doubt the Government is concerned with the costs of caring for an increasing number of adults whose illness could perhaps have been prevented. However, those caring for children would want to ensure that children have long and fulfilling lives, which, it is hoped, should provide the motivation to consider health promotion to be an important aspect of their role.

*Caring for Children and Families.* Edited by I. Peate and L. Whiting
© 2006 John Wiley & Sons Ltd

## HEALTH

It is important to consider what the word 'health' might mean. Everyone will hold different views about what health is. These views have been influenced by knowledge, past experiences and expectations. One person might consider health to be 'not being ill' while another person will consider themselves to be healthy if they can accomplish all the tasks they need to achieve. Health-care professionals may see health as the absence of disease or disability but for many people health is much more than this.

The World Health Organisation (WHO) has defined health as:

> a state of complete physical, mental and social well-being, not merely the absence of disease. (WHO, 1948, p. 100)

The ability to achieve complete well-being in each aspect of a person's life is perhaps rather idealistic, however this definition does indicate that health is much more than physical welfare.

Ewles and Simnett (1999) have identified a number of different dimensions within the concept of health; these demonstrate just how complex it is. Each of these will now be discussed in relation to child health.

*Physical health*   This concerns the mechanistic functioning of the body. The expectation for bodily functioning will vary according to the age of the child. For example, a 9-month-old who is unable to walk could have normal physical health, whereas a 5-year-old who is unable to walk may not be considered to be physically healthy.

*Mental health*   This is the ability to think clearly, which for children would include the ability to play and learn appropriately, according to their age.

*Emotional health*   This is the ability to express emotions such as fear, anger or joy in an appropriate manner. Once again, what is considered appropriate will vary with the age of the child or young person. A 2-year-old who lies on the floor and screams because he is angry at being refused a request for sweets is perhaps entirely normal, but a 13-year-old who behaves in a similar manner would not be considered to have behaved normally.

*Social health*   This is the ability to make and maintain relationships with other people. The types of relationships children make will vary with age. Young children are generally reliant on parents for their primary relationships, while teenagers would be expected to have a group of peers who are their friends.

*Spiritual health*   This may be connected with religious beliefs or it may be principles of behaviours and ways of achieving peace of mind. Young children are perhaps most likely to have beliefs similar to their parents, but as they grow older they will test these beliefs in order to formulate their own values.

*Societal health*  This recognises that a person's health is influenced by the environment, in which he or she is living. For example, a child who lives with parents who are unemployed, in a poor, rundown area of town would probably be less healthy than a child who lives with two working parents, in a more affluent part of town.

So far, the definitions of health that have been discussed are those proposed by adults; however, it is important to consider the views of children. Seedhouse (2001) proposes that health is a set of conditions that enable a person to achieve his or her realistic and chosen potential. This is helpful when considering children, as it recognises that there are factors that need to be present to enable children to achieve their potential. However, it is still an adult perspective of child health. So how do children view health? It is difficult for some children to define such an abstract term, but even young children have clear ideas about factors that influence their health and well-being. Consultations undertaken with children, young people and their families prior to the publication of *Every Child Matters* (Department for Education and Skills (DfES), 2003a) found that one of the five outcomes that mattered most was being healthy; this included enjoying good physical and mental health and living a healthy lifestyle.

It is apparent that children, from a young age, are aware of the importance of lifestyle and its impact on health; this was demonstrated in a study conducted by Oakley *et al.*, (1995). Children aged 9–10 years were asked to draw pictures of healthy and unhealthy factors in daily life. The largest category of factors implicated in health were those associated with diet, the second being exercise and sport. Children were also aware of unhealthy factors in the environment, including smoking, pollution and violence. Even younger children can identify aspects of the environment that affect their health; 4- and 5-year-olds living in Stepney (London) were able to draw and talk about issues impacting on their health (James, 1995); factors identified included:

- lack of safe outdoor play space
- fear of attack from dogs
- fear of abduction
- concern about the noise and smell of traffic.

**Activity**
*Think of a child you know. Make a list of different things that you think might impact on that child's health. Review the dimensions of health; these may prompt you to think of additional issues. You should have several on your list.*

It may be helpful to split the points you have identified into categories.

- You may have identified some that come from within the child, for instance is the child a girl or boy? Boys are more likely to be involved in accidents as will be discussed in Chapter 10.
- Each child is born with a unique genetic make-up which will impact on her or his health (e.g. some children have inherited tendencies to allergies, asthma and eczema).
- Other factors may come from the family into which the child is born. This might include how affluent the family is, the quality of care the child receives from the parents and what kind of food the family eats.
- A further area that influences child health is within the wider environment. This could include pollution or perhaps television advertising (this has a strong influence on child behaviours). The Government also has the potential to influence child health, which may be through publication of documents such as DH and DfES (2004), or the passing of laws that make it illegal to sell alcohol or cigarettes to young children.

If you have the opportunity to talk with a child you know, it might be interesting to ask them what things affect their health. Compare the child's ideas with your own.

## HEALTH PROMOTION

Thus far, this chapter has considered why child health is important, how child health might be defined and briefly considered issues that may impact on child health. So what is 'health promotion'? A most obvious answer is that it is improving a person's health. The WHO define it as:

> the process of enabling people to increase control over and improve their health.
> (WHO, 1984, p. 4)

This definition emphasises the importance of helping people to control their own health, rather than suggesting that it is something that can be done to people. In summary, health promotion is more than telling people what to do to improve their health. Tannahill (1985) suggests health promotion consists of three different types of activity:

- prevention
- health education
- health protection.

*Prevention*    This is generally understood to be any action that aims to stop ill health before it starts, but this is a limited view. Three levels of prevention have been identified: primary prevention aims to prevent the onset of disease, an example being immunisation. Secondary prevention aims to detect and cure a disease at an early stage before it causes irreversible problems, which might include stress management in schools. Tertiary prevention aims to minimise the effects of an already established disease, such as treatment for dental decay.

*Health protection* This makes healthier choices easier choices; this includes legislation that requires the wearing of seatbelts and forbidding the sale of alcohol to children.

*Health education* This is any activity which promotes health- or illness-related learning; an example could be teaching children how to brush their teeth. The scope of health promotion has been recognised by the DH and DfES (2004, p. 42) which states that:

> health promotion involves a range of activities at every level in society from government policies through local community strategies to individuals making healthy choices. (DH and DfES, 2004, p. 42)

In the past, health-promotion activities have often been directed at parents or carers, but it is important that the role of children and young people is also recognised. It has already been noted that young children are aware of factors that impact on their health; thus it seems reasonable that children should have the opportunity to participate in activities aimed at improving their health.

## PLANNING FOR HEALTH PROMOTION

Effective health promotion requires planning. The first stage in this process is to consider if there is a need for health promotion. It may be that a child or parent requests help in dealing with a specific issue, such as a mother asking advice about immunisations for her child. However, just because someone does not ask for help, it cannot be assumed there is not a need to help. Bradshaw (1972) recognised this and proposes four different types of need.

*Normative needs* These are defined by experts or professionals. This may result in a variety of opinions over what is a need; however, there are some standards over which there is agreement, for example the child health promotion programme offered by the DH and DfES (2004). Therefore, if a child has not been immunised according to the defined programme, a healthcare professional may perceive there is a need.

*Felt needs* These are what people feel they want (Ewles and Simnett, 1999). Perhaps a mother feels she wants more information about weaning her baby or a young person might wish to know how to avoid an unwanted pregnancy.

*Expressed needs* These are what people say they need. The mother might ask the health visitor for advice about weaning or the young person might go to a sexual health clinic. Not all felt needs are expressed, as might be the case if a young person is too embarrassed to go to a clinic or does not know where one is.

*Comparative needs*   These are defined in comparison to similar groups of people, some of whom are in receipt of health promotion and some of whom are not. If the young person seeking sexual health advice is unable to access a suitable clinic, but her cousin of the same age living in a neighbouring area is able to access such a service, there is a comparative need.

That identification of a need should lead to appropriate interventions to address that need.

---

**Activity**

*Gemma is 10 years old. She lives in a two-bedroomed flat with her mother and half brother James, aged 5 years. Gemma's father left home when she was a baby and she has not seen him for three years. Gemma's mother works part time in a local supermarket. Gemma has been admitted to the children's ward complaining of 'tummy pains'. Investigations have so far failed to iden- tify a physical cause for the pain, but Gemma has told one of the nurses that she hates school – no one likes her and the other children say that she is fat. The nurse has plotted Gemma's weight on a percentile chart; this has indi- cated that Gemma is slightly overweight. In addition, a student nurse who was helping Gemma to wash and dress has found that Gemma does not have a toothbrush in her wash bag, although she has been a patient on the ward for 24 hours.*

*What do you think are Gemma's health-promotion needs? How could Gemma be helped now and when she goes home?*

---

Within this situation you may have identified that:

- Gemma is slightly overweight;
- Gemma is unhappy at school and may be being bullied;
- Gemma's dental health may be poor.

You may have noticed that Gemma's apparent concern with her weight and perceived lack of popularity make these expressed needs. However, the lack of concern that she has no toothbrush would indicate a normative need. It would also be important to seek the views of Gemma's mother as any activ- ity may require her support. Each of the above issues will now be addressed, with some suggestions to improve Gemma's health.

## OVERWEIGHT AND OBESITY

'Overweight' is generally defined as exceeding an 'ideal' weight (Edlin *et al.*, 1996). Overweight and obesity are caused by consuming more calories than are being used in daily activity. Overweight could be considered to be the early stages of what might develop into obesity, although some authors use the terms interchangeably (Ruxton, 2004). In adults, body mass index (BMI) is used to identify those who are overweight and those who are obese. Adults are deemed overweight with a BMI of 25 kg/m$^2$ and obese at 30 kg/m$^2$, but children will be considered to be overweight or obese with different BMI measurements – these vary according to the age of the child (Fry, 2005). The DH, citing data from the Health Survey for England in 2002, found that being overweight and obese has increased by over 25% between 1995 and 2002, with a result that 28% of girls and 22% of boys aged 2–15 years could be placed in one of the categories. Therefore, Gemma is not alone. Obese children, and especially girls, are more likely to belong to lower socio-economic groups (DH, 2004a). Being overweight or obese can have long-term adverse affects on emotional well-being and self-esteem (Reilly et al., 2003). This would appear to be the case for Gemma. In addition, obesity increases the risk of adult ill health due to the increased likelihood of suffering from conditions such as coronary heart disease and type 2 diabetes. So what can be done to help Gemma?

The eating habits of children, which are often continued into adult life, are one factor that has resulted in the growing number of obese children and adults. If children are able to develop healthy eating habits, they will have a greater chance of a healthy adult life. Gemma spends a significant part of her day at school; therefore, it is important to consider how she can be helped to learn about healthy food choices at school. DH (2004a) and DfES/DH (2004) note that health-promotion activities are most effective when messages are coherent and consistent. This means that if children have lessons about healthy eating, the meals served in the dining room should also be healthy to enable children to put into practice what they have learnt. Of course, food served in the canteen is not the only food available in schools; so a food policy in Gemma's school could help her. This might mean that children are not allowed to bring carbonated drinks or chocolate to school and the tuck shop only sells fruit. This is an example of making healthier choices easier choices or health protection, since Gemma would have less opportunity to choose unhealthy food at school. Involving children in decisions about the kind of food served within the school could help children like Gemma; a school council could be set up to discuss menu options with the cook – this may facilitate behavioural change and help sustain the new lifestyle. After all, if Gemma wants to buy sweets or chocolate outside school, it is likely that she will have opportunities to do this and these will further increase as she grows older. The Government has stated that it wants to see schools 'actively promote healthy food and drink as part of an enjoyable and balanced diet and restrict the availability and promotion of other options' (DH, 2004a, p. 57).

It is important to note that schools may be constrained by a lack of resources. Time needs to be found within the constraints of the national curriculum, and appropriate personnel are required to teach the children. The finances of the school may also impact on the children's health as some schools receive additional funding through advertising and are reluctant to give up this source of income.

The school nurse could enhance the health of Gemma and her peers through provision of group sessions, perhaps focusing on healthy eating and exercise. One such activity in Hertfordshire is the Fit4Fun project, an after-school club for children aged 9–10 years, run by school nurses, which focuses on healthy eating and exercise (Hambleton, 2004). Children, parents and staff have been very positive about the project, many of the children stating that they had tasted food they had not previously tried. It is hoped that such schemes will soon be available to children throughout the UK as the Government has stated its intention to expand the role of the school nurse (DH, 2005).

In addition to school-based activities, Gemma needs the support of her family, as her mother is likely to provide many of her meals. Her mother may struggle to provide a healthy diet for Gemma. This could be due to lack of money, lack of time or a lack of knowledge about what is a healthy diet for children. According to DH (2000), British children are typically eating less than half the recommended five portions of fruit and vegetables per day, and one in five 4- to 18-year-olds eats no fruit at all during an average week. In addition, children growing up in low-income households eat less fruit and vegetables than those in higher-income households (DH, 2000). Gemma's mother could also be helped through school-based sessions focusing on healthy eating, assuming they are run at a time when she can attend. This is one activity that could be offered in the Extended Schools Programmes, which aim to make the school a force for health in every community.

While helping Gemma, it is also important to consider her brother. Perhaps he is not overweight now, but he may be at risk of becoming so. It is hoped that he is receiving fruit at school, as the National School Fruit Scheme entitles all infant children to a free piece of fruit each school day (DH, 2001). This could encourage him to try new fruits and establish a healthy eating pattern.

Although school might be the setting in which Gemma can be helped in the long term, it is important to consider what Gemma and her mother may learn about healthy eating while she is in hospital. The Health Care Commission's (2004) report states that:

> children's food did not have healthy options. Often there was only white bread, minimal vegetables and fruit, and too much kid's junk food like nuggets and waffles. (Health Care Commission, 2004, p. 11)

If this is the type of menu served to Gemma when in hospital, Gemma and her mother could be forgiven for thinking these kinds of food are recommended by healthcare professionals. While it is important that the opportunity for health promotion is not missed, the manner in which the diet is discussed is very important. Gemma's mother may be very worried about Gemma's hospitalisation and she may not be receptive to information about healthy eating; alternatively, she may feel that she is being criticised. If Gemma's mother needs further help, it may be appropriate to seek the support of a dietitian. Another less direct way to help Gemma might be through the use of notice boards or information racks within the ward that display health-promotion literature. This would then be available to her mother and, even if she does not want to discuss the issue, she would have a source of information for when she is ready.

Alongside healthy eating, exercise is important to prevent obesity. The DH (2004b) recommends that children participate in at least 60 minutes of moderate-intensity exercise per day. Physical exercise in childhood has a range of benefits including healthy growth and development, psychological well-being and social interaction (DH, 2004b), all of which are important to Gemma. As Gemma lives in a flat, her ability to participate in exercise may be limited. She could be encouraged to take part in physical activities at school, either during PE lessons or in after-school clubs, and perhaps even to walk to and from school. 'Fitbods', a project which started in Manchester in 1999, aimed to increase physical-activity levels among primary-school-aged children by implementing 'fun' games and activities in the playground at lunchtimes. Children received rewards for attendance; however, 81% of children said they would carry on without rewards. An evaluation conducted in 2002 reported 91% of children felt Fitbods had made them fitter and healthier (DH, 2003a).

As already discussed, the wider environment also has an impact on child health. For Gemma, this might be the impact of advertising on her eating habits. Even products marketed with a health-promotion message may not in themselves be healthy. In 2003, the *Guardian* reported a scheme called 'Cadbury get Active' in which children saved tokens from Cadbury's chocolate to earn sports equipment. It was calculated that a 10-year-old who ate enough chocolate to obtain a basket ball through the programme would need to play basketball for 90 hours to burn off the calories consumed (Lawrence, 2003). Thus, the initiative was not as 'health promoting' as it appeared at first glance.

## BULLYING

It is possible that Gemma is being bullied at school. In fact, this is quite likely as a recent survey found 51% of year 5 pupils reported that they had been bullied during the term, despite a requirement for all schools to have an anti-bullying policy (DfES, 2003b). Children within the study defined bullying to include verbal and physical abuse, theft, threatening behaviour and coercion. Bullying was felt to be any behaviour intended to cause distress or harm. Name-calling was the most prevalent form of bullying for year 5 pupils. Children who are overweight or obese have been found to be more likely to be victims of bullying (Janssen *et al.*, 2004). While children and young people identified a number of ways in which bullying might be tackled, great importance was attached to the involvement of pupils in decision-making at both an individual and school-wide level (DfES, 2003b). Children may wish to talk with adults about the situation, but they need to be given options regarding possible action. Therefore, Gemma needs the opportunity to talk through solutions, but she needs to feel she has some control over any action that may ensue. She may decide she does not wish any action to be taken, but she could seek support from websites such as Bullying Online (<http://www.bullying.co.uk>), which have been set up to provide advice and support for parents and children.

## DENTAL HEALTH

The student nurse who identified that Gemma does not have a toothbrush could talk to Gemma to see if she brushes her teeth regularly at home. The Children's Dental Health survey (National Statistics, 2003) found 75% of children said they brushed their teeth twice daily. However, the proportion of children who have plaque on their teeth has risen since 1993. Children from schools classed as deprived were more likely to have plaque (78%) as compared with children from non-deprived schools (70%). Walker (2000) found that children who lived with a single parent were less likely to report twice-daily tooth brushing, compared with those from two-parent families.

It is important that this opportunity for health promotion is not missed as Gemma and her mother may consider dental health to be unimportant. Toothbrushes should be available on the ward, and Gemma could be given one and encouraged to use it. The student nurse could explain to Gemma the importance of brushing her teeth, but Gemma cannot change the situation unless she has support from the adults around her. The student could discuss the need for Gemma to clean her teeth with her mother, but this needs to be done with great care. Gemma's mother may already be feeling quite vulnerable and it could appear that she is being criticised for the way she is caring for Gemma, implying that she is negligent. It is quite likely that a toothbrush was not a priority for Gemma's mother when Gemma was first admitted. This clearly demonstrates that any health-promotion activity needs to be implemented at an appropriate time, when the recipient is ready to receive the message.

In proposing some health-promotion activities to help Gemma and her family, you will have noted that some are conducted with individuals and some with groups. Some may be single sessions in which information is shared, while other activities are more long term. It is likely that the outcome of many of the approaches will not be evident for some time. If Gemma is able to improve her diet and activity level, some of the health-promotion benefits may not be seen until adult life, although it is hoped that an increase in her self-esteem would enhance her health in childhood and adolescence.

Thus far, health-promotion activities have focused upon a child who is able to be involved in at least some of the decisions regarding her health. What about promoting the health of a baby? What is the role of the healthcare professional and how far should it extend?

---

**Activity**

*Consider this situation:*

*Baby James is 2 months old and has been admitted to the ward with respiratory difficulties. James was born at 35 weeks' gestation (i.e. five weeks early) and is still very small (weighing 3 kg). His parents both smoke approximately 20 cigarettes a day. His mother, Jane, has told you that she started smoking when she was 14 years old and that she has smoked regularly for the last three years. She managed to reduce the number she smoked while she was pregnant, but as soon as James was born she returned to at least 20 cigarettes per day. She feels it would be difficult to give up as she is so worried about James.*

- *What should you do?*
- *A normative need has been identified but should action be taken now?*
- *What responsibility do you have to James?*
- *Do you have a responsibility to Jane?*

---

## SMOKING

Smoking is the single greatest cause of preventable illness and premature death in the UK. While there has been a small decline in the number of young people smoking since 2000, girls are more likely to be regular smokers. In 2004, 10% of girls and 7% of boys reported smoking regularly (Action on Smoking and Health (ASH), 2005). Eighty-two per cent of smokers take up the habit as teenagers, many going on to smoke all their lives (DH, 1998). Young people underestimate the addictive nature of smoking, believing they are in control and can stop smoking whenever they want (Andrews, 2004).

What can be done to reduce the chances of teenagers taking up smoking (Jane started smoking when she was 14 years old)? Schools may contribute through health education, in providing relevant information about the dangers of smoking. While education about the damaging health effects of smoking has been included in the curricula of most primary and secondary schools since the 1970s, this has not deterred many young people from starting the habit (ASH, 2005). Therefore, initiatives to prevent smoking in young people need to be developed in consultation with them. If the topic is addressed from an adult perspective, it is unlikely to appear relevant to the young person. Peer education could be used; this involves young people being trained as educators in order that they can share health information with others of a slightly younger age. Children and young people are more likely to take note of members of their peer group and, in addition, there are benefits to the peer educator as he or she gains new skills that should enhance confidence and self-esteem.

The Government has also endeavoured to deter young people from smoking by making it illegal to sell tobacco to anyone under 16 years of age. However, legislation alone is not sufficient to prevent tobacco sales to minors; it also requires compliance among retailers (ASH, 2005). This shows the impact of societal health on individuals. If the environment in which young people are growing up allows them easy access to health-damaging substances such as cigarettes, their health is more likely to be adversely affected. Advertising can also create the impression that smoking is a socially accepted norm, thus banning advertising at sporting venues can reduce the risk of young people taking up smoking.

Women who smoke while pregnant are likely to damage the health of their baby and to reduce the birth weight. What could have been done to help Jane stop smoking before James was conceived? Young people require different support systems from those of adults to help them stop smoking, and the provision of this type of support varies across the UK (Andrews, 2004). Some areas have provided specialist support for young people, facilitated by a network of NHS and non-NHS support. Even if such support does exist, it is important for it to be available at a time and place appropriate to young people, and they should know of its existence. Unfortunately, it appears that this may not have happened for Jane.

So what can be done to help James? It is estimated that 17000 hospital admissions, in a single year, of children under 5 years of age are due to their parents' smoking; additionally, 25% of cot deaths could be caused by mothers smoking (DH, 1998). Children of parents who smoke are more likely to develop asthma; it could be argued that James has the right to a smoke-free atmosphere. When children aged 7–10 years were asked, 82% disliked adults smoking near them (DH, 2003b). Since James is too young to assert the right to smoke-free air for himself, it falls to responsible adults to do it for him. However, how far should you go to protect James and what is acceptable activity on the part of the Government?

Article 8 of the Human Rights Act (1998) states:

> Everyone has the right to respect for his private and family life, his home and his correspondence.

Therefore, it could be argued that Jane has the right to live her life the way she has chosen, without interference.

The Government has stated that it does have a responsibility to protect children from tobacco. One activity within a campaign to raise awareness of the damaging effect that smoking in the house has on children was the distribution of bibs with a 'Second-hand Smoking' slogan – these were given to every baby

born in December 2003 (DH, 2003b). This coincided with a television adver-
tisement featuring the slogan 'If you smoke, I smoke.' To some this might seem
entirely acceptable, while to others the message may be a little too direct and
it could cause distress to some families. For this reason, when promoting health,
it is important to consider ethical principles and how they relate to practice.

## THE APPLICATION OF ETHICAL PRINCIPLES

### BENEFICENCE AND NON-MALEFICENCE

'Beneficence' and 'non-maleficence' require the health promoter to do good
and avoid harm. However, there is potential for conflict in trying to do good
and not harm. The distribution of bibs with a 'Second-hand Smoking' slogan
was intended to do good to babies in encouraging adults not to smoke.
However, for some families this may have provoked conflict if one parent
smoked while the other did not; alternatively, a mother might have been very
distressed if she had smoked in the past and a previous child had suffered a
cot death. For some parents who are living in difficult circumstances, smoking
is one way to maintain their mental health, and encouraging them to stop
smoking could lead to a decreased ability to cope with their children.

### AUTONOMY

Autonomy means having the right to determine how one lives one's life. Therefore, it could be argued that the healthcare professional has no right to interfere in Jane's life and to suggest that she stops smoking, since it is the choice
that she has made. However, does Jane have all the relevant information to
make an informed choice? Jane should at least be made aware of the risks,
but should an attempt be made to persuade Jane to give up smoking? It
could be argued that James needs someone to advocate on his behalf since he
cannot do it for himself. What if the healthcare professional also smokes? The
person has the right to determine her or his own life, but it may not be appropriate to tell Jane smoking is harmful to James, when smelling of smoke
oneself.

### JUSTICE

In order to ensure justice, decisions need to be made about allocation of time
and resources. It would be unfair if someone spent all day with Jane encouraging her to stop smoking if this compromised the care of other children on
the ward. Equally, provision of numerous smoking-cessation support groups
at the expense of other resources, such as sexual health clinics, could be unfair.
Therefore, resources need to be provided on the basis of need.

## EXPLORING THE ROLE OF THE HEALTHCARE PROFESSIONAL

If it is decided that the opportunity to promote health for Jane and James should be taken, one approach that could be used is an empowering one-to-one encounter as described by Tones and Green (2004):

### THE COMMUNICATION PHASE

The communication phase enables the establishment of a rapport with Jane. To achieve this, it is important to actively listen to Jane's concerns about her baby. Jane may then be given some information about the risks of smoking to babies.

### THE MOTIVATION PHASE

The motivation phase necessitates the identification of Jane's feelings about that information, checking whether she has understood it and if she intends to do anything about it. There may also be discussion about why Jane smokes and factors that prevent her giving up; consideration may be given to whether now is the most appropriate time to stop smoking. It may be that the shock of an admission is a trigger to encourage Jane to change her lifestyle, but it may be she is just too stressed to even think about it. Even if she can't stop, a compromise or 'contract' could be made, perhaps reducing the number smoked each day.

### THE SUPPORT PHASE

The support phase provides support to sustain the choice. It may not be possible to provide long-term support, thus the need for multidisciplinary working. Jane may be given details of local smoking-cessation groups, and even if this information is not available a member of the multidisciplinary team could speak with Jane's health visitor or practice nurse to ensure continued support when James is discharged home.

## EVALUATING HEALTH-PROMOTION ACTIVITIES

Evaluation occurs when a judgement is made about the value of an activity – in this case health promotion. A judgement might be made about the outcome of an activity (that is what has been achieved) and/or the process of an activity (that is how it was achieved) (Ewles and Simnett, 1999). Evaluation is important as it can help to improve practice and justify the use of resources required. However, for many health-promotion activities the outcome may not be apparent for some time afterwards; as has already been mentioned, the outcomes for Gemma may not be evident for many years. Despite this, the process of the activity can be judged; consideration can be given to whether a good relationship was established with Gemma and her mother, whether they listened to what was said and whether they seemed interested. If the activity went well, the factors that made it successful can be identified. These aspects of the health promotion can be judged as the activity is occurring and reflected upon afterwards.

For James, once again, long-term outcomes are important, but the process is also significant. Was a relationship built with Jane that enabled her to share her concerns about her smoking? If so, how was it achieved? The answers to these questions may then inform future health promotion with other parents who smoke.

## CONCLUSION

This chapter has considered child health and child health promotion. Scenarios have been provided to illustrate some of the key concepts within health-promotion practice. However, these are only examples of possible situations when health promotion would be of value to the child and her or his family. There are many more opportunities for health promotion within both hospital and community settings. It is important that health promotion is viewed as an integral part of your role in order that children are afforded the maximum potential for a happy and healthy life, both now and as they grow into adult life.

## REFERENCES

Action on Smoking and Health (2005) *Young people and smoking – Fact sheet 3* <http://www.ash.org.uk> (accessed 23 March 2005).

Andrews S (2004) The challenge of teenage smoking. *Nursing Times* 100(6), 52–53.

Bradshaw JR (1972) The taxonomy of social need. In: McLachlan G (ed) *Problems and Progress in Medical Care*. Oxford: Oxford University Press.

Department of Health (DH) (1998) *Smoking Kills: a White Paper on tobacco*. London: DH.

Department of Health (DH) (2000) *National Diet and Nutrition Survey: Young people aged 4–18 years*. London: DH.

Department of Health (DH) (2001) *The National School Fruit Scheme: Evaluation summary*. London: DH.

Department of Health (2003a) *Fitbods* <http://www.doh.gov.uk/cmo/innovations/fitbods.htm> (accessed 12 May 2003).

Department of Health (DH) (2003b) *New Secondhand Smoke Bibs for Every Baby Born in December*. <hhtp://www.dh.gov.uk/PublicationsAndStatistics/Pressreleases/PressreleasesNotices/fs/> (accessed 10 December 2004).

Department of Health (DH) (2004a) *Choosing Health*. London: DH.

Department of Health (DH) (2004b) *At Least Five a Week: Evidence on the impact of physical activity and its relationship to health*. London: DH.

Department of Health (DH) (2005) *Choosing Better Health: A food and diet action plan*. London: DH.

Department for Education and Skills (DfES) (2003a) *Every Child Matters*. London: DfES.

Department for Education and Skills (DfES) (2003b) *Tackling Bullying: Listening to the views of children and young people*. London: DfES.

Department for Education and Skills (DfES) (2004) *Starting Early: Food and nutrition education of young children*. London: Ofsted Publication Centre.

Department for Education and Skills & Department of Health (DfES/DH) (2004) *National Service Framework for Children, Young People and Maternity Services: Supporting local delivery*. London: DfES/DH.

Department of Health & Department for Education and Skills (DH/DfES) (2004) *National Service Framework for Children, Young People and Maternity Services: Core standards*. London: DH/DfES.

Edlin G, Golanty R and McCormack Brown K (1996) *Health and Wellness* (5th edn). Sudbury, MA: Jones & Bartlett Publishers.

Ewles L and Simnett I (1999) *Promoting Health: A practical guide* (4th edn). London: Balliere Tindall.

Fry T (2005) How to identify obesity in children – and when. *Practice Nursing* 16(1), 25–29.

Hambleton H (2004) Fit4fun. *Community Practitioner* 77(10), 367–368.

Health Care Commission (2004) *Patient Survey Report: Young patients*. Oxford: Picker Institute, Europe.

James J (1995) Children speak out about health. *Primary Health Care* 5(10), 8–12.

Janssen I, Craig W, Boyce W and Pickett W (2004) Associations between overweight and obesity with bullying behaviours in school-aged children. *Pediatrics* 113(5), 1187–1194.

Lawrence F (2003) How much chocolate do you need to eat to get a free netball? The *Guardian* <http://education.guardian.co.uk/schools/story/0,5500,945533,00.html> (accessed 29 April 2003).

National Statistics (2003) Children's Dental Health National Statistics Online <http://www.statistics.gov.uk.cci/nugget_print.asp?ID=975> (accessed 14 December 2004).

Oakley A, Bendelow G, Barnes J, Buchanan M and Nasseem Husain O (1995) Health and cancer: Knowledge and beliefs of children and young people. *British Medical Journal* 310(6986), 1029–1033.

Reilly J, Methven E, McDowell Z, Hacking B, Alexander D, Stewart L *et al.* (2003) Health consequences of obesity. *Archives of Disease in Childhood* 88(9), 748–752.

Ruxton C (2004) Obesity in children. *Nursing Standard* 18(20), 47–52, 54–55.

Seedhouse D (2001) *Health: The foundations for achievement* (2nd edn). Chichester: John Wiley & Sons.

Tannahill A (1985) What is health promotion? *Health Education Journal* 44(4), 167–168.

Tones K and Green J (2004) *Health Promotion: Planning and strategies*. London: SAGE.

Walker A (2000) *National Diet and Nutrition Survey: Young people aged 4–18 years: Volume 2: Report of the oral health survey*. London: TSO.

World Health Organisation (WHO) (1948) *Preamble to the Constitution of the World Health Organisation as Adopted by the International Health Conference*, New York, 19–22 June, 1946; signed on 22 July 1946 by the representatives of 61 States (Official Records of the World Health Organisation, No. 2, p. 100) and entered into force on 7 April 1948. Geneva: WHO.

World Health Organisation (WHO) (1984) *Health Promotion: A discussion document on the concept and principles*. Copenhagen: WHO.

# 6  Biological Aspects of Child Health Care

## P. HARWOOD

## INTRODUCTION

The aim of this chapter is to explore the related anatomical, physiological and biological aspects that influence health and altered physiology in children. Topics discussed include:

- the structure and function of the circulatory system and some common congenital disorders in children;
- the structure and function of the respiratory system and some common childhood respiratory disorders;
- temperature regulation and febrile convulsions;
- the structure and function of the digestive tract, and some health problems encountered by children;
- the structure and function of the eye and ear and related disorders.

Throughout the chapter the reader is presented with review questions to enable you to check your understanding as you work through some of the issues. Each review question is provided with suggested responses.

## THE CIRCULATORY SYSTEM

The main function of the circulatory system is to transport oxygen and nutrients to all parts of the body and to remove waste products. Oxygen is vital as it is required for energy production in all body cells. The circulatory system is made up of the heart and blood vessels (Shier *et al.*, 2004). The blood vessels consist of arteries, arterioles, capillaries, venules and veins. (See Table 6.1 and Figures 6.1 and 6.2 for differences between arteries and veins.)

### CAPILLARIES

Capillaries are made up of thin endothelium only one cell thick and have a very small lumen. This facilitates diffusion or movement of oxygen and nutri-

*Caring for Children and Families*. Edited by I. Peate and L. Whiting
© 2006 John Wiley & Sons Ltd

**Table 6.1** Differences between arteries and veins

| Arteries | Veins |
| --- | --- |
| Normally carry oxygenated blood away from the heart. | Normally carry deoxygenated blood back to the heart. |
| Blood within the arteries is under pressure; they are strong, thick and elastic. | Blood is at a lower pressure, walls are not as thick and have a larger lumen to help blood flow. |
| They have no valves since the pressure is high. | They have valves to ensure that blood flows in the right direction. |

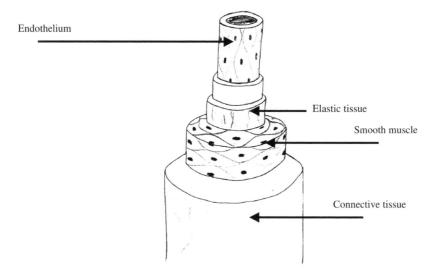

**Figure 6.1** Diagram of an artery.

ents to the tissues and carbon dioxide and waste products from the tissues into the blood for removal as waste products.

## THE ANATOMY OF THE HEART

The heart is a muscular organ whose main function is to pump blood throughout the body. It is made up of four chambers (Saladin and Wysenberg, 2001), the upper left and right atria and the lower left and right ventricles. The two atria receive blood returning to the heart through veins. The right atrium receives *deoxygenated* blood from the upper and lower parts of the body to the heart, and the left atrium receives *oxygenated* blood from the lungs. (Figure 6.3).

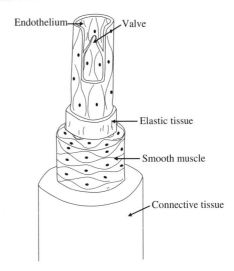

**Figure 6.2** Diagram of a vein.

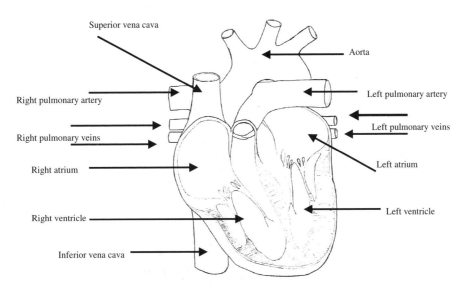

**Figure 6.3** Diagram of the heart.

**Review question**

*What is deoxygenated blood?*

> Deoxygenated means that it has low oxygen levels since most of the oxygen
> has been given up to the tissues.

Ventricles are the lower chambers that pump blood away from the heart. The
right ventricle pumps deoxygenated blood to the lungs (pulmonary circulation), and the left ventricle pumps oxygenated blood to the upper and lower
parts of the body (systemic circulation) (Neil and Knowles, 2004) (Figure 6.4).

**Review question**

*Briefly summarise blood flow through the heart*

> Deoxygenated blood high in carbon dioxide flows from the body through
> the *superior* and *inferior vena cavae* to the *right atrium* and is pumped to
> the *right ventricle* through the *tricuspid valve*. From the right ventricle it is
> pumped through the *pulmonary artery* to the lungs for oxygenation. From
> the lungs oxygenated blood flows through the *pulmonary veins* into the *left
> atrium*. From the left atrium it is pumped into the *left ventricle* through the
> *bicuspid (mitral valve)*. From the left ventricle it is pumped through the
> *aorta* to the rest of the body (Shier *et al.*, 2004) (Figure 6.4).

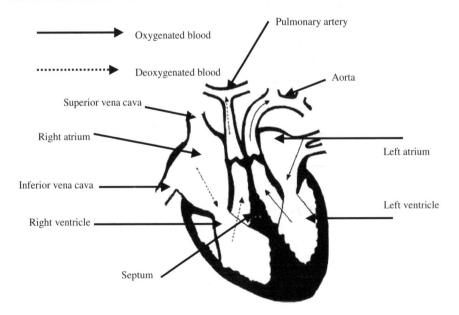

**Figure 6.4** Blood flow though the heart.

THE PUMPING ACTION OF THE HEART

**Systole**

Contraction of the cardiac muscle in the ventricles marks the beginning of *systole*. When ventricles contract, blood from the left ventricle is forced into the aorta; at the same time blood from the right ventricle is forced into the pulmonary artery. This creates an increase in pressure within the aorta and systemic circulation known as *systolic blood pressure*.

**Diastole**

Relaxation of the cardiac muscle marks the beginning of *diastole*. This decrease in arterial pressure is known as *diastolic blood pressure*.

**Review question**

*What pressures are noted when measuring blood pressure?*

> When measuring blood pressure, the *systolic* and *diastolic* pressures are detected.

Blood pressure ranges with age. The blood pressure measurements are also affected by the child's condition.

ELECTRICAL ACTIVITY OF THE HEART

Heart muscle cells are interconnected so that an impulse originating in one cell can spread to neighbouring cells, causing the whole heart to contract. The heart also contains pacemaker cells that can generate a rhythmic contraction of muscle. When the electrical activity of the heart is disrupted, this can result in abnormal heart beats, which are detected by an electrocardiogram (ECG). This can be displayed on paper, as occurs when an ECG machine is used, or on a monitor.

Normal heart rates vary depending on the child's age and stage of development.

DEVELOPMENTAL ISSUES

The heart and blood vessels develop from 4 to 8 weeks of gestation (Wong *et al.*, 2003). Overall foetal circulation is at a relatively higher pressure known as *high vascular resistance*. During intra-uterine circulation, there are special structures which are present. These include the *foramen ovale*, which connects the right and left atrium. The foramen ovale is expected to close soon after birth, but in some situations this does not occur creating what is often referred to as a 'hole' in the heart.

**Table 6.2** Acyanotic and cyanotic congenital abnormalities of the heart

| Acyanotic | Cyanotic |
| --- | --- |
| atrial septal defect, ventricular septal defect, patent ductus arteriosus, coarctation of the aorta | transposition of great arteries, tetralogy of Fallot |

## CONGENITAL HEART DEFECTS

These occur when a child is born with a heart-related problem. The defect may affect the heart, the great vessels or both (Ryan *et al.*, 2003). Congenital heart defects can be *cyanotic* or *acyanotic*. 'Cyanotic' means that there is a blue discoloration of the skin and mucous membranes due to lack of oxygen. 'Acyanotic' means that no blue (cyanotic) discoloration is present (Table 6.2).

## ACYANOTIC HEART DEFECTS

There are a number of acyanotic congenital heart defects; the most common ones are discussed below.

### Atrial septal defect (ASD)

This occurs when there is a 'hole' in the heart connecting the atria or upper chambers. Because the pressure in the left atrium is higher than in the right atrium, blood is forced into the right atrium creating a pressure which increases blood flow to the lungs causing pulmonary hypertension (high blood pressure within the vessels of the lungs). This can also cause abnormal rhythms of the heart. The severity of the condition is related to the size of the 'hole'. If the pressure in the right atrium is prolonged, this can lead to an enlargement of the right atrium.

### Ventricular septal defect (VSD)

When a 'hole' in the heart connects the ventricles, a VSD is present. Blood is forced from a high-pressure area into an area of lower pressure which is from the left ventricle to right ventricle. The increase in blood flow can result in increased blood flow to the lungs. An increase in blood circulating to the lungs can lead to frequent respiratory infections and an enlargement of the heart. Very large defects can lead to heart failure (Woolf *et al.*, 2002).

### Patent ductus arteriosus (PDA)

During foetal development, there is a passageway (ductus arteriosus) connecting the aorta and the pulmonary artery. In this situation blood is channelled away from the unexpanded lungs. This often closes in 1–2 days after birth (Woolf *et al.*, 2002). If this fails to close, the infant is said to have a *patent ductus arteriosus*. Because the aorta has a much higher pressure than the pulmonary artery, blood is shunted from the aorta to the pulmonary artery increasing pulmonary blood flow. Increased pulmonary pressure can ultimately lead to heart failure.

## CYANOTIC HEART DEFECTS

In cyanotic heart defects, oxygenated blood mixes with deoxygenated blood and enters the systemic circulation. The child presents with cyanosis. Examples of cyanotic heart defects are listed below.

### Tetralogy of Fallot

This defect consists of four abnormalities. These include:

- ventricular septal defect (VSD);
- pulmonary valve stenosis (narrowing);
- overriding aorta (aorta slightly displaced towards the right ventricle overriding the VSD);
- right ventricular hypertrophy (enlargement) (Wong *et al.*, 2003).

The child presents with cyanosis, the degree of which depends on the severity of obstruction of blood flow from the right ventricle into the pulmonary artery.

### Transposition of great arteries

In this abnormality, the aorta arises from the right ventricle and the pulmonary artery from the left ventricle. As there is a reversal of the great arteries, the aorta pumps deoxygenated blood to the rest of the body, and the pulmonary artery pumps oxygenated blood to the lungs. Survival is impossible unless there is another existing abnormality mixing oxygenated and deoxygenated blood (for example PDA).

## THE RESPIRATORY SYSTEM

The main function of the respiratory system is to supply oxygen to the body cells and to remove carbon dioxide. Oxygen is needed for energy production, and carbon dioxide is the end product of *energy production* also referred to as *metabolism*. Structurally, the respiratory system is made up of air passages which consist of the upper and lower respiratory tracts.

## UPPER RESPIRATORY TRACT

The upper respiratory tract conducts air into the lungs, also purifying and humidifying the air. This tract is made up of the nostrils, nasal cavity, pharynx, larynx and trachea.

*Nostrils* Also called *nares*, their function is to take in air from the atmosphere. Air is important in that it contains oxygen which is required for energy production, essential for the maintenance of life. Neonates are obligatory nose breathers (Markenson, 2002), hence nasal secretions can cause airway obstruction. 'Obligatory' means that they breathe mainly through their nose and do not adapt to mouth breathing.

*Nasal cavity* The main function of the nasal cavity is to filter and humidify air. The respiratory tract contains tiny hairs known as *cilia*. Their main function is to filter any dust or tiny particles that may be inhaled with air, hence purifying the inhaled air. The upper region of the nasal cavity contains smell receptors (Marieb, 2004).

*Pharynx* The pharynx is located at the back of the nose. The pharynx is a common passageway for both air (*nasopharynx*) and food (*oropharynx*), which explains why it is easy to have airway obstruction caused by food particles. Sharing the same passageway makes it possible to breathe from both the nose and mouth. The pharynx also contains *tonsils* which are an organ of the immune system.

*Larynx* This is made up of cartilage and contains the *epiglottis*, which consists of a small flap of tissue that prevents food and fluid from entering the trachea during the process of swallowing. The larynx also contains vocal chords which vibrate and produce sound.

*Trachea* This contains smooth muscle supported by cartilage. Cartilage keeps the trachea open.

**Review question**

*Why is it essential to give humidified oxygen?*

> Prolonged administration of oxygen can result in a dry mucous membrane (Ashurst, 1995).

The trachea divides to form two primary *bronchi*.

## LOWER RESPIRATORY TRACT

The lower respiratory tract is made up of the bronchi and bronchioles and the lungs. The bronchi divide into *bronchioles* which end in the *alveoli*, tiny sacs found in the lung tissue. (See Figure 6.5 for a diagrammatic presentation of the respiratory tract.)

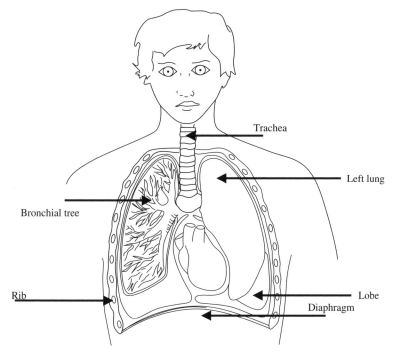

**Figure 6.5** Diagram of the respiratory tract.

## Review question

*Why are the alveoli important?*

> Each alveolus is surrounded by a network of capillaries, which are branches of the pulmonary artery containing deoxygenated blood received by the heart from the rest of the body. The alveoli and capillaries are single layered, and this facilitates the exchange of oxygen and carbon dioxide by the process of *diffusion* (Figure 6.6).

*'Diffusion'* is the movement of particles from an area of high concentration to a low concentration until there is equilibrium (Figure 6.7).

Oxygen moves into the pulmonary capillaries and is transported to the heart, which pumps the oxygenated blood to the rest of the body tissues. Carbon dioxide moves into the alveoli and is exhaled during expiration. Oxygen is carried mainly by haemoglobin (Hb) in the red blood cells, which is why it is important to have a normal range of haemoglobin. The oxygen rich blood is transported to the heart where it is pumped to the rest of the body.

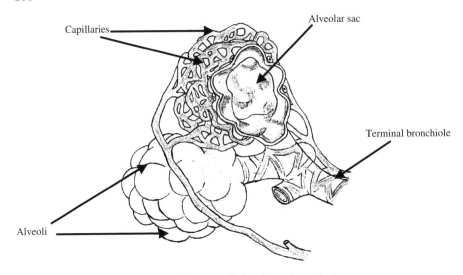

**Figure 6.6** Diagram of alveoli and capillaries.

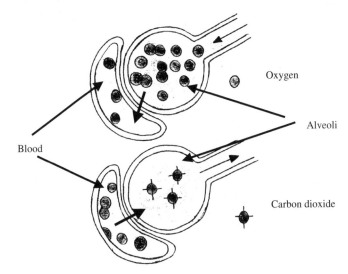

**Figure 6.7** Diagram of simple diffusion.

## Review question

*Why is a child with anaemia lethargic?*

Because there is less haemoglobin in the blood. Haemoglobin carries oxygen to the tissues for energy production.

**Review question**

*Where does carbon dioxide come from and why do the lungs get rid of it?*

---

In the presence of oxygen and glucose, body cells produce energy, and carbon dioxide is a by-product. However, carbon dioxide is an 'acid gas'. Accumulation of carbon dioxide makes blood more acidic (acidosis), which can interfere with essential body functions.

---

**The process of breathing**

*'Inspiration'* is the process of taking air into the lungs and *expiration* is breathing out. The major muscle of breathing is the *diaphragm*, which is dome-shaped. It separates the chest from the abdomen. It is an important muscle in that it contracts and moves downwards expanding the chest cavity, a process essential for drawing in air into the lungs (*inspiration*). The diaphragm is innervated by the *phrenic nerve*. Infants use the diaphragm as the main muscle of respiration (Markenson, 2002), hence the importance of observing the abdomen when assessing respiration.

The *intercostal* muscles located between the ribs are also involved in the process of breathing. During inspiration, they contract and move the ribs upwards and outwards, facilitating the process of inspiration by increasing the size of the chest cavity. This creates a negative pressure which sucks air into the lungs. The intercostal muscles are innervated by the *intercostal nerve*. During expiration, the diaphragm relaxes and moves upwards, reducing the size of the chest cavity creating a positive pressure, which pushes air out of the lungs. Expiration is normally passive as it does not require muscle contraction.

Overall control of ventilation is by the respiratory centre in the *medulla*. Anatomical differences in children of different ages result in age-related normal respiratory rates.

## WHY ARE CHILDREN DIFFERENT FROM ADULTS?

In infants and young children:

- the tongue is relatively large;
- the chest wall is cartilaginous and compliant and the airways are narrow (Helms, 2000), hence the ease with which airway obstruction can occur;
- there is less alveolar surface area for gaseous exchange;
- respiration can be irregular and *apnoea* can occur in early infancy and preterm babies (apnoea is a condition where the baby temporarily stops breathing);
- surfactant production is reduced in preterm babies.

*Surfactant* is produced by alveolar epithelium. It reduces surface tension (Chamley *et al.*, 2005). It helps to keep alveoli open since lungs collapse without surfactant, and if this happens the baby is unable to breathe. This can occur in a condition known as *respiratory distress syndrome* (RDS). RDS is a disorder of prematurity which occurs due to insufficient concentrations of surfactant. These infants may require artificial ventilation and replacement of surfactant.

**Use of accessory muscles**

Children use the sternocleidomastoid muscle resulting in 'head bobbing', a sign of increased work of breathing (Jevon *et al.*, 2004).

## SYMPTOMS OF RESPIRATORY PROBLEMS

The common symptoms of respiratory problems include:

- *Coryza*, which is a runny blocked nose that can be accompanied by *sneezing*.
- *Cough*, a mechanism that helps clear respiratory passages. Coughing occurs because of an accumulation of secretions or presence of an irritant which stimulates the cough reflex. A cough can be dry or productive, producing sputum. Sputum can be mucoid, which is clear and white. It can also be watery and frothy as happens if the child has pulmonary oedema. Infection can produce yellow or green sputum. In some instances blood can be present (haemoptysis).
- *Breathlessness* is another symptom of respiratory problems. It can present as *dyspnoea*, a sense of breathlessness, or as *orthopnoea*, which is difficulty in breathing when lying flat. The child is nursed upright to prevent the contents of the abdomen from compressing the diaphragm.

*Cyanosis* occurs when there is bluish discoloration of the skin or mucous membrane due to a lack of oxygen. Signs of respiratory distress include:

- tachypnoea (an increase in respiratory rate)
- irritability
- cyanosis not relieved by oxygen
- tachycardia (an increase in heart rate)
- wheezing, which is a sound produced by narrowed airways as in asthma; this is produced mainly during expiration
- stridor: a harsh whistling sound produced mainly during inspiration as seen in croup
- an increase in the work of breathing
  - recession
  - nasal flaring (Dieckmann *et al.*, 2000)
  - tracheal tug
  - grunting
  - use of accessory muscles
  - stridor/wheeze
  - head bobbing – a sign of dyspnoea in an exhausted or sleeping child
- fatigue.

## ALTERATIONS OF THE UPPER RESPIRATORY TRACT

### Epiglottitis

Inflammation of the epiglottis often presents as a sore throat, fever and an inspiratory stridor. This condition can be a medical emergency as the child can present with an airway obstruction due to inflammation. It is frequently caused by a bacterial organism known as *Haemophylus influenzae* type *B* (Woolf *et al.*, 2002). The disorder occurs more frequently during the winter months.

### Laryngotracheobronchitis (croup)

This is a laryngotracheal infection due to parainfluenza virus or respiratory syncitial virus (O'Callagan and Stephenson, 1992). This is marked by inflammation and increased mucosal secretion of the larynx, trachea and bronchi, often resulting in airway obstruction. Laryngotracheobronchitis often affects children from 6 months to 4 years (Lissaeur and Clayden, 2003) and is common during the winter months. Croup often presents with a hoarse voice and stridor accompanied by a barking cough.

## ALTERATIONS OF THE LOWER RESPIRATORY TRACT

### Bronchiolitis

Bronchiolitis is a viral inflammation of the bronchioles. The most common cause is the *respiratory syncitial virus*. The infection is transmitted by droplet infection. It often affects infants of 1–9 months of age and is rare after the age of 1 year (Lissaeur and Clayden, 2003). The infection is common during winter months and the infant often presents with a harsh cough, difficulty in feeding and symptoms of respiratory distress.

## CHRONIC RESPIRATORY PROBLEMS

### Asthma

Asthma is a chronic reversible inflammatory disorder of the airways leading to airway obstruction owing to airway oedema, increased mucus secretion and bronchial smooth muscle spasm (McCance and Huether, 2006), which causes a narrowing of the airways also known as *bronchoconstriction*. It is characterised by episodes of wheezing, cough and a feeling of tightness in the chest. *Extrinsic* asthma affects children of any age and is a common disease of childhood. It is often induced by extrinsic factors such as dust mites or pollen which can be identified and avoided where possible. Extrinsic asthma can be associated with atopy, hay fever and eczema. *Intrinsic* asthma often occurs in adults and does not tend to have identifiable triggers.

**Review question**

*What are the extrinsic triggers of asthma in children?*

---

Asthma can occur as a result of an allergic reaction, which may be triggered by allergens such as:

- dust mites
- pollen
- animal fur
- fungus
- dust
- cigarette smoke
- cold air
- food
- exercise

---

**Review question**

*What are the symptoms during an asthma attack?*

---

- wheeze and a cough
- increased work of breathing (nasal flaring and intercostal recession)
- a pronged expiratory phase which can be accompanied by a wheeze
- decreased air movement detected during auscultation
- cyanosis

---

**Peak expiratory flow rate (PEFR)**

This is a measure of the maximum *expiratory flow rate* during forced expiration using a peak flow meter following a full inspiration (Ayres and Turpin, 1997). It is measured in litres per minute and the results are based on the age, sex and height of the child. It is a cheap non-invasive way of detecting limitations of air flow, which can be easily performed at home. The procedure can also be used before and after medication to objectively assess its effectiveness. However, very young children are unable to use this technique.

**Aims of treatment**

These are to maintain oxygenation, reverse symptoms, reduce asthma attacks and maintain adequate pulmonary function. It is also essential to avoid 'triggers'.

## DISORDERS OF THE IMMUNE SYSTEM

Children with compromised immunity often present with recurrent infection, chronic infection and/or incomplete clearing of infection. In immunodeficiency diseases, the immune system is underdeveloped or it is blocked (Martini *et al.*, 2004).

### SEVERE COMBINED IMMUNODEFICIENCY (SCID)

This is a group of disorders which result in deficiency of both cell mediated and humoral immunity – this often occurs during the first month of life. The child frequently presents with a history of chronic infection, recurrent chest infections (for example *Haemophylus influenzae*) and unusual infection (for example *Pseudomonas aeruginosa*) (Ryan *et al.*, 2003).

### HIV AND AIDS

HIV (human immunodeficiency virus) is caused by a human immunodeficiency virus, and the terminal stage of this process is known as AIDS (acquired immunodeficiency syndrome) (McCance and Huether, 2006). In newborn babies, this can be caused by vertical transmission from an infected mother. Infection can also occur during delivery or postnatally through breast feeding. Breast feeding by women infected with the HIV virus is considered a high-risk factor for transmission of HIV (Philip, 1996). For the same reason, breast feeding is not recommended for an infected mother. In the older child, transmission can occur through infected blood or blood products. The infant or child with HIV presents with symptoms of immunodeficiency, which include recurrent respiratory infections and diarrhoea. Failure to thrive is also present.

### ANAPHYLAXIS

This occurs due to an exaggerated immune system response which usually affects hypersensitive individuals. Anaphylaxis is systemic affecting mast cells throughout the body (Martini *et al.*, 2004). Causes of anaphylaxis can include ingested substances as seen in peanut allergy or other food allergies, or when a substance is injected, as seen in bee stings. The symptoms of anaphylaxis can occur immediately, resulting in hypovolaemia and shock or they can be delayed. Anaphylaxis can also present with urticarial rash or a feeling of being warm. Skin reactions are often the first sign. A child may also complain of a feeling of uneasiness and restlessness, irritability and disorientation (Wong *et al.*, 2003). Facial swelling, tachycardia, hypotension, pallor and a wheeze can follow. Anaphylaxis is a medical emergency, and help must be summoned promptly.

**Temperature regulation**

The body's temperature is maintained at a relatively constant level in spite of changes in ambient temperatures and alterations in heat production due to metabolism and activity. This is essential because enzymes which control metabolic processes work within a very narrow temperature range. Metabolism is the sum of all the physical and chemical events that release and use energy in order to maintain life. Babies have relatively higher metabolic rates and a 3-month-old baby's normal body temperature is 37.5 °C. Metabolism decreases with age and by 13 years the normal body temperature is 36.6 °C (Wong *et al.*, 2003). In order to maintain a constant body temperature, the amount of heat lost must be equal to heat gained.

**Heat generation**

Heat is constantly generated by muscles and the liver which generate energy through chemical activities which produce heat, a process that involves metabolism. The higher the metabolic rate, the greater the amount of heat generated. Young children have a higher metabolic rate (Casey, 2000), hence their ability to produce heat rapidly. Digestion involves contraction of muscles, and this also produces a significant amount of energy. Heat can also be produced by shivering. Thyroxine is a hormone that generates heat through an increase in cellular metabolism (Montague *et al.*, 2005).

**Heat loss**

Most heat is lost through the skin and the remainder is lost in expired air, urine and faeces. Babies and young children have a relatively larger surface area to volume ratio, hence their ability to lose heat rapidly (Hazinski, 1992). They are not well insulated as they have a thin layer of subcutaneous fat (McCance and Huether, 2006).

**Review question**

*Why is it important to cover a baby's head in an effort to conserve heat?*

> The head constitutes a relatively larger surface area ratio, hence the effectiveness of covering the head.

Heat loss is affected by environmental temperature, hence the importance of maintaining a neutral thermal environment. A neutral thermal environment is an environment that minimises the use of oxygen consumption and use of calories while maintaining a normal core temperature (Wong *et al.*, 2003).

When the body temperature is elevated, receptors from the skin and internal organs send impulses to the thermoregulatory centre of the hypothalamus (heat-generating centre), which is a thermostatic set point located at the base of the brain. The brain activates heat-losing mechanisms, which include peripheral vasodilation and sweating. During vasodilation, more blood flows through the blood vessels and heat is lost by conduction, convection and radiation (Martini *et al.*, 2004).

## Conduction

Loss of heat directly into cooler objects through direct contact.

## Convection

Loss of heat through the air. Air heated by the body rises and is replaced by cooler air.

## Radiation

This involves energy lost in infrared heat waves (Montague *et al.*, 2005). Heat is lost from the warmer body to the cooler environment, and most body heat is lost in this way.

## Evaporation

When sweating, heat is lost through evaporation. Heat needed for evaporation is contained in the skin. Prolonged excessive sweating can lead to dehydration and electrolyte imbalance.

Other methods of losing heat include loss through expired air. Conscious measures include removing excess clothing and creating a cooler environment. Babies and young children rely upon adults, hence the importance of detecting environmental temperature changes.

## Review question

*Identify two causes of a raised body temperature in a child*

1. infection
2. prolonged exposure to very high heat as in heat stroke

When the body temperature falls below normal levels (hypothermia), heat-producing mechanisms are activated and these include shivering, which generates heat. Skin blood vessels constrict and this decreases the amount of heat lost. Babies cannot shiver and rely on an increase in brown adipose tissue, which is a highly vascularised heat-producing (thermogenic) tissue. This process is also known as 'non-shivering thermogenesis'. Brown adipose tissue has a high content of cell mitochondria (Chamley *et al.*, 2005), which are involved in the generation of energy. This increase in metabolism requires oxygen and noradrenaline (norepinephrine) secreted by sympathetic nerve endings.

**Review question**

*Why is it important to increase calorific intake in a child with hypothermia?*

In order to meet the increase in metabolism required to generate heat.

**Fever**

Fever is present when the body temperature is elevated above 37.5 °C (Porth, 1994). During the presence of a fever, the hypothalamic set point is elevated by *interleukin 1* (also known as an *endogenous pyrogen*) (Shier *et al.*, 2004), which is produced when the body is invaded by micro-organisms. This is carried to a part of the brain known as the *hypothalamus*, which responds by resetting the temperature control point to a higher level. The brain responds by stimulating heat-producing mechanisms and skeletal muscles are activated to increase heat production. At the same time, sweating is decreased and blood flow to the skin is reduced. As a result, the body temperature increases as fever develops. Elevation of the body temperature helps the immune response combat infection (Thibodeau and Patton, 2005).

**Review question**

*Explain why an increase in fluid intake is recommended when caring for a child with a high body temperature*

A child with a fever requires an increased fluid intake (Shier *et al.*, 2004) since fluid is lost through sweating.

**Febrile convulsions**

A febrile convulsion is a seizure that is associated with the development of a fever. No other cause is found and it is not associated with meningitis (Lissaeur and Clayden, 2003). Febrile convulsions often occur in young children from 6 months to 5 years and are associated with a fever. Convulsions rarely occur after the age of 5 years. Parents are often concerned about the possibility of the development of epilepsy. This anxiety must be allayed as 98% of these children will not develop epilepsy or any neurological damage (Wong *et al.*, 2003).

The development of a fever stimulates the hypothalamus to initiate heat-losing mechanisms. However, in children under 5 years, the heat-losing centre is immature and can cause convulsions when stimulated (Moules and Ramsay, 1998).

**Review question**

*Identify two ways of reducing fever in practice*

1. fanning
2. giving prescribed antipyretics

## THE DIGESTIVE SYSTEM

The main function of the digestive system is ingestion, digestion, absorption and elimination. The digestive processes include *ingestion*, the process of taking in food, *propulsion*, which is movement of food aided by peristalsis, *mechanical digestion*, which is the physical breakdown of food, *chemical digestion*, in which food is broken down by enzymes, and *absorption* and *defecation* (Marieb, 2004) (Figure 6.8). Absorption is the movement of the products of digestion from the lumen of the gut into the blood or lymph (Marieb, 2004) and defecation is the elimination of materials as faeces (Martini *et al.*, 2004).

The components of the digestive system include the mouth, teeth, oesophagus, stomach, duodenum, small and large intestines, the rectum and the anus. Accessory organs of digestion include the salivary glands, the liver and the pancreas. Accessory organs are not situated within the digestive tract and provide enzymes and substances that aid the digestive process.

### The mouth

In the mouth, food is chewed, mixed with saliva and is made up into a bolus for easy swallowing. Saliva contains *salivary amylase*, which starts the digestion of carbohydrates.

Reflexes that are present at birth include sucking, swallowing and the gag reflex. Sucking can be nutritive or non-nutritive. Non-nutritive sucking occurs in newborn babies and is not associated with nutrition. It is said to be for satisfying the basic sucking urge (Wong *et al.*, 2003).

### The teeth

Deciduous or milk teeth erupt within the first two years of life. *In utero*, the development of teeth occurs during the fifth month of gestation. For the same reason, the nutritional status of the mother can affect the child's teeth devel-

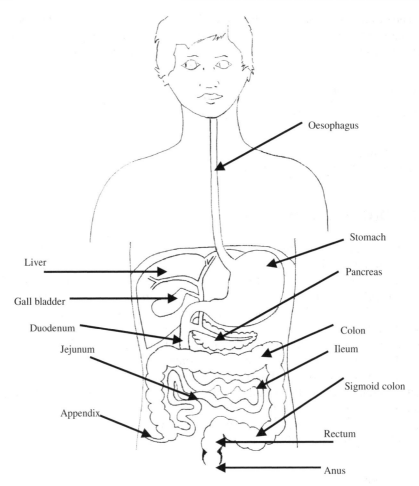

**Figure 6.8** Diagram of the digestive tract.

opment. The first tooth can erupt at about six months of age; however, there are individual differences. 'Teething' is a term used to describe tooth eruption. It can be associated with red, swollen and sensitive gums. Drooling can also be present, but this is mainly associated with the development of salivary glands (Schulte *et al.*, 1997).

## The oesophagus

This is a muscular tube which directs food from the mouth to the stomach mainly by peristalsis.

## The stomach

The stomach is a C-shaped tube which churns food using its muscular walls. It secretes hydrochloric acid, which provides the optimum pH for digestive enzymes to work as these enzymes require an acid medium for optimum functioning. Hydrochloric acid also has a protective function in that it kills ingested bacteria. Cells within the stomach also secrete the enzyme *pepsinogen* which is converted to *pepsin*, an enzyme that digests proteins.

### Functions of the stomach

- storage of food;
- mechanical digestion by churning peristaltic waves that mix food with gastric juice and propel it into the duodenum;
- chemical digestion of proteins by pepsin;
- absorption (Marieb, 2004).

## ACCESSORY ORGANS OF DIGESTION

### The pancreas

The pancreas produces bicarbonate-rich pancreatic enzymes. These enzymes include *amylase* for the digestion of carbohydrates, *lipase* for the digestion of fat and *proteases* for the digestion of proteins. The pancreas is also an endocrine gland which produces insulin.

### The liver

The liver produces bile which is a yellow/green alkaline solution that emulsifies fats. Bile is stored in the gall bladder. The liver stores glucose as glycogen, which is converted back to glucose when required.

### The small intestine

The major divisions of the small intestine are the *duodenum, jejunum* and *ileum*. The duodenum is joined by the pancreatic duct and common bile duct from the liver. The pancreatic duct can be blocked by thick mucus secretions in children with cystic fibrosis, hence the need for a substitute for pancreatic enzymes.

The main functions of the small intestine include:

- completion of digestion of fat, carbohydrate and proteins
- absorption by the intestinal villi.

### The large intestine

This is composed of the *caecum* with the *appendix* attached to it. It also consists of the ascending, transverse and descending colon, sigmoid colon, rectum and anal canal. Its main function is to reabsorb water and some electrolytes and vitamins (vitamin K) (Marieb, 2004).

'Defecation' is the process of removing waste or indigested substances, including cellulose that is not broken down by human digestive enzymes. Cellulose creates the bulk essential in preventing constipation. Defecation is triggered by a full rectum and involves the parasympathetic nervous system, which aids the contraction of the rectal walls.

## MALNUTRITION

This occurs when there is an imbalance between the supply of nutrients and the body's demand for them to ensure adequate growth (World Health Organisation (WHO), 2000). An adequate supply of protein is essential in order to provide amino acids and enzymes. Carbohydrate is essential for energy production.

Malnutrition can be due to an inadequate food intake or failure to absorb or utilise nutrients. Chronic illnesses affecting the digestive system can lead to impaired digestion or absorption. Malnutrition affects physical growth, cognitive development and can also compromise the immune system.

### Review question

*Give two examples of childhood chronic illnesses that can lead to malnutrition*

Cystic fibrosis due to lack of digestive enzymes and chronic diarrhoea resulting in poor absorption.

Malnutrition can also be associated with lack of micronutrients, which include vitamins and minerals. (See Table 6.3, which identifies vitamins, their source and function.)

### Vitamin deficiencies

Vitamins are organic compounds required for growth and good health. Small amounts are required (Marieb, 2004) (Table 6.4).

Minerals are also required for smooth functioning of the body (Table 6.5).

### Disorders of the alimentary canal

#### Cleft lip

This occurs when there is a failure of fusion of embryonic structures of the face. One or both sides of the lip can be separated (Wong, 2003). This defor-

**Table 6.3** Vitamins, their source and function

| Vitamin | Source | Function |
|---|---|---|
| A (retinol) | carotene found in deep-yellow and deep-green vegetables, fish liver oils | synthesis of photoreceptor pigments found in the retina |
| B | leafy green vegetables, whole grain | part of coenzyme required for energy production |
| C (ascorbic acid) | citrus fruits and leafy vegetables | antioxidant |
| D | produced by the skin in the presence of light, fish liver oils, eggs | mobilises calcium for bones |
| E | wheat germ and vegetable oils, dark-green leafy vegetables | antioxidant |
| K | leafy green vegetables, synthesised by bacteria in large intestines | required for blood clotting |

**Table 6.4** Signs of vitamin deficiency

| Vitamin | Signs and symptoms of deficiency |
|---|---|
| A | night blindness, hair changes |
| B | loss of appetite, scaly skin |
| C (ascorbic acid) | poor healing of wounds and increased susceptibility to infection |
| D | rickets and poor growth |
| Folic acid | anaemia, can affect development of the neural tube *in utero* resulting in neural tube defects |

**Table 6.5** Minerals and their function

| Mineral | Function |
|---|---|
| calcium | bones and teeth |
| chloride | osmotic pressure and pH of body fluids |
| sulphur | protein synthesis |
| potassium | muscle contraction, transmission and conduction of nerve impulses, maintenance of normal cardiac rhythm |
| sodium | maintenance of extracellular osmotic pressure; essential for nerve impulse transmission, and muscle contraction |
| iron | formation of red blood cells |

mity occurs during rapid foetal development. The cleft often occurs below the nostril and can affect the nasal cartilage and septum. The deformity can be mild or severe, and sometimes a cleft lip and palate can be present together.

*Cleft palate*

The palate forms the roof of the mouth and is made up of the soft and hard palate. The hard palate is made of bone, and the soft palate consists of tissue. A cleft palate is an opening in the roof of the mouth. It can present as an incomplete cleft, involving the uvula and soft palate, or complete cleft, involving the hard palate and nostril. Cleft palate is more common in females (Woolf *et al.*, 2002). Children with a cleft lip and palate can present with feeding and speech difficulty.

*Oesophageal atresia*

This involves failure of the oesophagus to reach the stomach. It often ends as a blind pouch. Children with this disorder can present with a *tracheo-oesophageal fistula*, which is an opening between the oesophagus and the trachea. This is usually identified during the infant's first feed which can trigger a cough as food enters the lungs. In severe cases, cyanosis may also be present.

*Gastro-oesophageal reflux*

This is due to an incompetent oesophageal sphincter which allows stomach contents to reflux into the oesophagus. This is often aggravated by lying flat or by a full stomach. Because the contents of the stomach are acid, they can erode the lining of the oesophagus leading to inflammation (oesophagitis).

*Hypertrophic pyloric stenosis*

Hypertrophic pyloric stenosis is a congenital progressive hypertrophy of the muscles of the pyloric sphincter causing partial or complete obstruction. The infant presents with projectile vomiting during or immediately after feeds, hunger, dehydration and weight loss (Chamley *et al.*, 2005). The symptoms often present two to three weeks after birth. The infants are often irritable because they are hungry. If vomiting is severe, fluid and electrolyte imbalances can occur. Corrective surgery is performed (Ramstedt's operation), which involves splitting of pyloric muscle.

**Diarrhoea**

This is characterised by an increase in frequency or decrease in consistency of stools. Diarrhoea can be classified as infectious or non-infectious. It can also be classified as acute or chronic.

*Infectious diarrhoea*

Diarrhoea can be caused by bacterial infections such as *Escherichia coli* (*E. coli*) and *salmonella* (Table 6.6). Parasites such as *Giardia lamblia* can also

**Table 6.6** Causes of diarrhoea

| Infectious | Non-infectious |
|---|---|
| **Bacterial:** | food allergy |
| *Salmonella* | metabolic disorders: |
| | • coeliac disease |
| | • cystic fibrosis |
| *Escherichia coli* | disaccharide deficiencies |
| *Shigella* | infant overfeeding |
| *Campylobacter jejuni* | faecal overflow |
| **Protozoal:** | |
| *Giardia lamblia* | |
| *Cryptosporidium* | |
| **Fungal:** | |
| *Candida albicans* | |

cause diarrhoea, which is the commonest cause of chronic diarrhoea in children. This is often associated with malabsorption, especially of fat and carbohydrates. The characteristic stools are offensive and there is weight loss and abdominal distension. Some infants develop lactose intolerance following infectious diarrhoea (Chamley *et al.*, 2005).

*Non-infectious factors*

Non infectious causes of diarrhoea include malabsorption syndromes such as coeliac disease and cystic fibrosis, food allergy and lactose intolerance. These disorders cause chronic diarrhoea (Wong *et al.*, 2003). Overfeeding with carbohydrates can lead to diarrhoea since indigested carbohydrate can create an osmotic pressure which draws fluid into the gut and this increases the amount of water lost as stools.

Diarrhoea can lead to a loss of fluid resulting in dehydration.

*Dehydration*

An infant has a relatively higher metabolic rate compared to children and adults, hence fluid requirement is larger *per kilogram body weight*. In a healthy child, there must be a balance between fluid gain and fluid loss in order to maintain homeostasis. When fluid loss exceeds fluid gain, the child becomes dehydrated. One of the major causes of dehydration in children is diarrhoea and vomiting (Advanced Life Support Group (ALSG), 1997). Infants have a higher distribution of extracellular fluid compared to children and adults. Extracellular fluid is easily lost compared to intracellular fluid, hence infants have a higher risk of developing dehydration (Hazinski, 1992). Dehydration may be accompanied by electrolyte imbalances. If a fever is present, the metabolic rate is increased and more water is lost through sweating. A child with rapid respirations will also lose water (Schulte *et al.*, 1997).

Dehydration can be classified as *isotonic, hypotonic* or *hypertonic* (Willock and Jewkes, 2000). The classifications are made according to the amount of sodium lost, which depends on the amount of fluid and electrolytes lost.

In isotonic dehydration, an equal amount of fluid and electrolytes is lost. When intravenous fluids are given, the sodium concentration is similar to that of plasma (isotonic). Whereas, in hypotonic dehydration, more sodium is lost and the plasma sodium concentration is low. Hypertonic dehydration occurs because more water is lost and the plasma concentrations of sodium are elevated. This is often associated with gastroenteritis and can also present in a child with diabetes insipidus.

## Elimination

### Constipation

Constipation is difficulty, delay or pain during defecation (Buchanan, 1992). Constipation can be caused by an alteration of stool consistency or the motility of the colon (Arce *et al.*, 2002). At some time during childhood, 34% of children suffer from constipation (Muir and Burnett, 1999). Lack of dietary fibre, dehydration or lack of exercise can cause constipation. Some drugs such as morphine or codeine can also cause constipation. In Hirshsprung's disease, constipation is present from birth due to poor innervation of the bowel and upper parts of the colon (Staiano *et al.*, 1999). As a result, there is poor propulsion of faecal material into the rectum, and it is often associated with abdominal distension. Some children with constipation have faecal incontinence or soiling.

## COMMUNICATING

### THE EAR

#### Structure of the ear

The ear is an organ of hearing and balance. It is made up of three parts: the *external ear*, the *middle ear* and the *internal* (inner) *ear* (Figure 6.9). The function of the external and middle ear is to conduct sound waves, whereas the inner ear is for hearing and balance.

### The external ear

This is made up of the *auricle*, or pinna, the *external auditory meatus* and the *tympanic membrane*. The pinna is made up of cartilage. Its main function is to collect sound waves and direct them to the external auditory meatus or ear canal

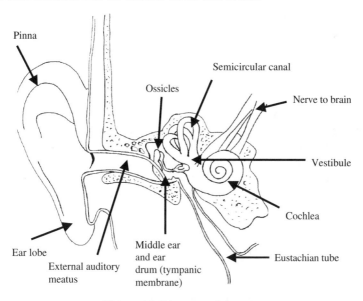

**Figure 6.9** Diagram of the ear.

towards the tympanic membrane. The skin of the ear canal is covered with tiny hairs and contains sebaceous glands which open into the hair follicles.

The auditory meatus is a tube which connects the pinna to the tympanic membrane (ear drum). It is made up of the cartilaginous portion and the osseous portion. The cartilaginous portion contains ceruminous glands that are modified sweat glands (Martini *et al.*, 2004), which secrete wax (cerumen). Wax is protective in that it traps foreign particles such as dust. The canal also contains hairs for protection.

*The middle ear*

This section contains air and is connected to the *nasopharynx* through the *Eustachian tube*. The main function of the Eustachian tube is to equalise air pressure between the middle ear and atmospheric air. Inequalities in pressure can lead to hearing difficulties. Air on both sides of the tympanic membrane facilitates vibration of the ossicles by sound waves. The pressure in the middle ear must equal the pressure of atmospheric air.

**Review question**

*While travelling on a train, a child complains of deafness as the train is going through a tunnel. Explain why this occurs*

This occurs due to inequalities in air pressure.

The *tympanic membrane*, or ear drum, separates the outer ear from the middle ear. It consists of thin, semi-transparent connective tissue. Externally it is covered by skin and internally by mucous membrane. When sound vibrates the ear drum, it is transmitted into the middle ear. The middle ear contains three ossicles – the *malleus, incus* and *stapes* – which are very small bones. Their function is to transmit sound from the ear drum to the cochlea in the inner ear. From the cochlea sound is transmitted to the brain.

The malleus is positioned next to the ear drum and is shaped like a hammer. The incus is shaped like an anvil, and the stapes is shaped like a stirrup and its base fits into the *fenestra vestibule* (oval window). The ossicles are stabilised by fine ligaments and are covered by mucous membrane. The inner ear also contains nerves that transmit impulses associated with balance.

## HEARING LOSS IN CHILDHOOD

Hearing loss can be:

- **conductive** – usually due to disorders of the outer and middle ear;
- **sensorineural** – due to damage of the cochlear nerve;
- **mixed** – involving both conductive and sensorineural.

Conductive deafness can be alleviated by surgical intervention. However, damage to the cochlear nerve involves loss of nerve hair cells from the organ of Corti and is usually permanent. Other causes of deafness include maternal rubella, wax, a foreign body and traumatic perforation of the ear drum (Dhillon and East, 1994).

### Otitis media

Otitis media is inflammation and oedema of the middle ear. In children this often follows a respiratory tract infection, allergic rhinitis or hypertrophic adenoids (Moules and Ramsay, 1998). The inflammatory process can be associated with secretion of fluid by the cells in the middle ear, blocking the Eustachian tube. The fluid becomes thick and glue-like, a condition known as 'glue ear' (Woolf *et al.*, 2002). The accumulation of fluid in the middle ear prevents the ossicles from vibrating effectively (Letko, 1992), causing hearing impairment. This can interfere with the child's speech development, hence the importance of early detection and intervention.

Surgical intervention involves grommet insertion which is done through an incision made in the tympanic membrane (myringotomy). Grommets relieve fluid build-up and facilitate aeration of the middle ear. If blockage of the Eustachian tube is due to hypertrophy of the adenoids, adenoidectomy may be performed (Campbell and Glasper, 1995).

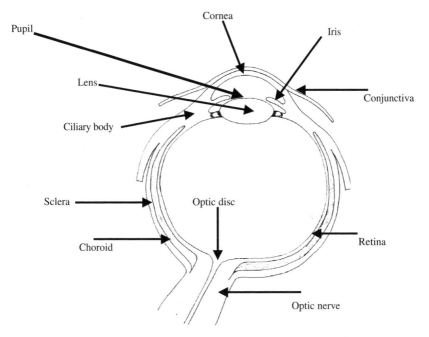

**Figure 6.10** Diagram of the eye.

## THE EYE

The eye is an organ of vision with visual receptors linked to the brain by nerves (Figure 6.10). It lies in a bony orbit of the skull for protection.

Features of the eye:

- The *outer fibrous* layer known as the sclera or white of the eye, which is made up of collagenous and elastic fibres that protect and maintain the shape of the eye. In front of the eye (anteriorly), the sclera becomes a clear transparent membrane known as the *cornea*. The cornea is clear because it contains a few cells and no blood vessels. The transparency of the membrane facilitates entry of light into the retina of the eye.

- The *choroid* is the middle vascular layer. It contains a brown pigment *melanin*, hence its brownish-black appearance. Light from the retina is absorbed by melanin. The *ciliary body* is an extension of the choroid. It is situated anteriorly, and gives attachment to *suspensory ligaments*, which hold the lens in position. Contraction and relaxation of the ciliary muscle alters the shape of the lens. The lens is biconvex and transparent. The function of the *lens* is to bend light in order to focus it on to the retina of the eye. In order to see close objects, the lens thickens, a process known as *accommodation*, needed for clear vision. The space in front of the lens contains aqueous fluid (humour), and the space behind the lens contains vitreous humour. The fluids maintain the shape of the eye.

- The *iris* is the coloured part of the eye which extends from the ciliary body. It is situated between the cornea and the lens. The iris also contains brown pigment. The amount of pigment determines eye colour: if there is a lot of pigment present, the eyes are brown-coloured; however, if the amount is reduced, the eyes are blue-coloured. Newborn babies have bluish eyes because the pigment is not yet developed (Chamley *et al.*, 2005).
- The *pupil* is an opening in the centre of the iris. It allows light to enter the eye and also controls the amount of light entering the eye. Contraction of circular muscles constricts the pupil and is often associated with bright light. Contraction of radial muscles dilates the pupil associated with poor lighting.
- The *retina* is the inner layer made up of visual photoreceptors known as *rods* and *cones*. Cones are for coloured vision, whereas rods are for colour-less vision. *Rhodopsin* is the light-sensitive pigment in rods. It produces reactions that activate nerve impulses through the optic nerve (second cranial nerve). The photoreceptors require vitamin A, and this is stored by the retina. There is an area of the retina that has no receptors and there is no vision. This is known as the 'blind' spot.

### Accessory organs of the eye

Accessory organs of the eye include the lachrymal glands, which secrete tears. *Lachrymal ducts* also transport tears into the nasal cavity. Tears have a protective function since they reduce friction and remove debris, preventing bacterial infections and providing oxygen and nutrients to parts of the conjunctiva (Martini *et al.*, 2004). They also contain an enzyme known as *lysozyme* with antibacterial properties.

*The conjuctiva*   This is a mucous membrane which lines the inner surface of eyelids. The conjuctiva is constantly bathed by tears.

*Extrinsic muscles*   These move the eye in order to follow a moving object.

## COMMON EYE DISORDERS IN CHILDREN

### Watery and sticky eyes

This is often due to naso-lachrymal gland obstruction in the newborn. It usually occurs during the first couple of weeks of life, and often resolves spontaneously (Robinson and Roberton, 1999).

## Conjunctivitis

Conjunctivitis is inflammation of the conjunctiva. This can be due to bacterial or viral infection, allergies or irritating chemicals. The child with conjunctivitis often presents with a 'pink eye'.

## Cataracts

Cataracts present with opacity of the lens of the eyes.

## Diplopia

Diplopia is double vision, which can be caused by a dysfunction of ocular muscles which occurs in strabismus.

## Myopia

Myopia is short-sightedness. The affected child has the ability to see close objects clearly but is unable to see distant objects.

## Glaucoma

This occurs when there is an increase in intra-occular pressure. In infancy, this often presents with a cloudy and enlarged cornea and photophobia. Constant increased pressure can damage the optic nerve resulting in blindness.

## Strabismus (squint)

This may be due to an abnormality of the nervous system supplying the eye muscle, resulting in weak muscles of the affected eye and misalignment. In children prompt treatment is required as it can result in *amblyopia*, a reduction in vision (McCance and Huether, 2002).

## CHAPTER SUMMARY

### CIRCULATORY SYSTEM

- The function of the circulatory system is to transport *oxygen* and *nutrients* to all parts of the body, and to remove *waste products*.
- It is made up of the *heart* and *blood vessels*.
- The foetal circulatory system contains openings or ducts that close soon after birth. In some instances these do not close, resulting in congenital abnormalities of the heart. These can be *cyanotic* or *acyanotic*.

## THE RESPIRATORY SYSTEM

- The main function of the respiratory system is to supply *oxygen* to the tissues with the help of the circulatory system and to get rid of *carbon dioxide*.
- It consists of the *upper respiratory tract*, which conducts and purifies air, and the *lower respiratory tract*, which facilitates diffusion of oxygen into the systemic circulation and carbon dioxide from the blood into the alveoli of the lungs for removal from the body by the lungs.
- Alterations of the upper respiratory tract include *epiglottitis* and *laryngotracheobronchitis*, which can cause obstruction of air flow.
- Alterations of the lower respiratory tract include *bronchiolitis* and *asthma*, which can also cause airway obstruction.

## DISORDERS OF THE IMMUNE SYSTEM

- Disorders of the immune system include *severe combined immunodeficiency* (SCID) and HIV/AIDS, which is due to a human immunodeficiency virus. Both conditions present with symptoms caused by a compromised immune system.

## MAINTAINING BODY TEMPERATURE

- The body maintains a constant body temperature through *heat-generating* and *heat-losing* mechanisms.
- When heat-losing mechanisms slow down or when metabolism is increased, a child presents with a *fever*.
- When heat-losing mechanisms are enhanced, or metabolism slows down, a child presents with *hypothermia*.

## THE DIGESTIVE SYSTEM

- The main functions of the digestive system are associated with *ingestion*, *digestion*, *absorption* and *elimination*.
- The digestive system is composed of the *mouth*, teeth, oesophagus, stomach, small intestine and large intestine. *Accessory organs* lie outside the digestive tract and provide enzymes, which are substances that aid the digestive process. These include the *salivary glands*, the *liver* and the *pancreas*.
- *Malnutrition* can occur due to *inadequate food intake* or *failure to absorb or utilise* nutrients.
- *Vitamins* and *minerals* are essential for the growth and functioning of the body.
- Disorders of the digestive system include cleft lip, cleft palate, oesophageal atresia, gastro-oesophageal reflux and hypertrophic pyloric stenosis.
- *Diarrhoea* can result in dehydration and electrolyte imbalance.
- *Constipation* is passage of dry, infrequent stools.

## THE EAR

- The ear is an organ of *hearing* and *balance*. It is made up of the external, middle and inner ear.
- The *external* and *middle ear* are made up of structures that facilitate *transmission* of sound into the inner ear.
- The *internal ear* perceives sound and is also involved with *balance*.
- Hearing loss in childhood can be *conductive, sensorineural* or *mixed*.
- *Otitis media* is inflammation of the ear which can result in exudation of fluid causing 'glue ear', which can interfere with hearing.

## THE EYE

- The eye is made up of the outer fibrous layer known as the *sclera*, the middle vascular layer (*choroid*) and the *retina*.
- Common eye disorders include *conjunctivitis, cataracts, diplopia, myopia, glaucoma* and *strabismus*.

## REFERENCES

Advanced Life Support Group (ALSG) (1997) *Advanced Paediatric Life Support: The Practical Approach* (2nd edn). London: BMJ Publishing Group.

Arce DA, Ermocilla CA and Costa H (2002) Evaluation of constipation. *American Family Physician* 65(11), 2283–2288.

Ashurst S (1995) Clinical: Oxygen therapy. *British Journal of Nursing* 4(9), 508–514.

Ayres J and Turpin P (1997) *Peak Flow Measurement*. London: Chapman & Hall.

Buchanan A (1992) *Children who soil: Assessment and treatment*. London: John Wiley & Sons.

Campbell S and Glasper EA (1995) *Whaley and Wong's Children Nursing*. London: Mosby.

Casey G (2000) Fever management in children. *Nursing Standard* 14(40), 36–40.

Chamley CA, Carson P, Randall D and Sandwell M (2005) *Developmental Anatomy and Physiology of Children*. Edinburgh: Elsevier.

Dhillon RS and East CA (1994) *Ear, Nose and Throat and Head and Neck Surgery 1*. London: Churchill Medical Communication.

Dieckmann R, Brownstein D and Gausche-Hill M (2000) *American Academy of Pediatrics: Pediatric education for pre-hospital professionals*. Boston: Jones & Bartlett Publishers.

Hazinski MF (1992) *Nursing Care of the Critically ill Child* (2nd edn). St Louis: Mosby.

Helms P (2000) The respiratory system. In: Haddard DF, Greene SA, Olver RE and Chantler C (eds) *Core Paediatrics and Child Health*. London: Churchill Livingstone.

Jevon P, Soanes K, Berry K, Pearson GA and Beattie T (2004) *Paediatric Advanced Life Support: A practical guide*. Edinburgh: Butterworth-Heinemann.

Letko M (1992) Detecting and preventing infant hearing loss. *Neonatal Network* 11(5), 33–38.

Lissauer T and Clayden G (2003) *Illustrated Textbook of Paediatrics* (2nd edn). Edinburgh: Mosby.

Marieb EN (2004) *Human Anatomy and Physiology* (6th edn). San Francisco: Pearson/Benjamin Cummings.

Markenson DS (2002) *Pediatric Prehospital Care.* Englewood Cliffs, NJ: Prentice Hall.

Martini FN, Ober WC, Garrison CW, Welch KW, Hutchings RT and Ireland KI (2004) *Fundamentals of Anatomy and Physiology* (6th edn). Englewood Cliffs, NJ: Prentice Hall.

McCance KL and Huether SE (2006) *Pathophysiology: The biologic basis for disease in adults and children* (5th edn). St Louis: Mosby.

Montague SE, Watson R and Herbert R (2005) *Physiology for Nursing Practice.* Edinburgh: Elsevier.

Moules T and Ramsay J (1998) *Children's Nursing.* Cheltenham: Stanley Thornes.

Muir J and Burnett C (1999) Setting up a nurse-led clinic for intractable childhood constipation. *British Journal of Community Nursing* 4(8), 395–399.

Neil S and Knowles H (2004) *The Biology of Child health: A reader in development and assessment.* London: Palgrave.

O'Callagan C and Stephenson T (1992) *Pocket Paediatrics.* London: Churchill Livingstone.

Philip AGS (1996) *Neonatology: A practical guide* (4th edn). Philadelphia: WB Saunders.

Porth M (1994) *Pathophysiology: Concept of altered health states* (4th edn). Philadelphia: Lippincott-Raven.

Robinson MJ and Roberton DM (1999) *Practical Paediatrics* (4th edn). Edinburgh: Churchill Livingstone.

Ryan S, Gregg J and Patel L (2003) *Core Paediatrics: A problem-solving approach.* London: Arnold Publishers.

Saladin KS and Wysenberg DV (2001) *Anatomy and Physiology: The unit of form and function* (2nd edn). Boston: McGraw-Hill Higher Education.

Schulte EB, Price DL and Ames SR (1997) *Thompson's Paediatric Nursing: An introductory text.* Philadelphia: WB Saunders.

Shier D, Butler J and Lewis R (2004) *Hole's Human Anatomy and Physiology* (10th edn). New York: McGraw Hill.

Staiano A, Santoro L, De Marco R, Miele E, Fiorillo F, Auricchio A *et al.* (1999) Autonomic dysfunction in children with Hirshprung's disease. *Digestive Diseases and Sciences* 44(5), 960–965.

Thibodeau GA and Patton GA (2005) *The Human Body in Health and Disease* (4th edn). St Louis: Elsevier Mosby.

Willock J and Jewkes F (2000) Making sense of fluid balance in children. *Paediatric Nursing* 12(7), 37–42.

World Health Organisation (WHO) (2000) *Malnutrition: The global picture.* Geneva: WHO.

Wong DL (1999) *Whaley and Wong's Nursing Care of Infants and Children* (6th edn). St Louis: Mosby.

Wong DL, Hockenberry MJ, Wilson D, Winkelstein ML and Kline NE (2003) *Wong's Nursing Care of Infants and Children* (7th edn). St Louis: Mosby.

Woolf N, Wotherspoon A, Young M (2002) *Essentials of Pathology.* London: Elsevier.

# 7 Assessment and Monitoring of Children

**L. GORMLEY-FLEMING**

## INTRODUCTION

Accurate assessment of the child, interpretation of data and implementing care based on assessment are essential skills for the nurse. It is the first part of the nursing process (Figure 7.1). Without assessment, the nurse cannot begin to formulate a picture of the child's and family's needs. The nurse's primary aim should be to care for the child who is ill rather than the illness itself, thus gathering information that is unique to them and information that will help to identify the child's and family's actual and potential health problems. Assessment of the child takes place in both the hospital and community setting. The skill remains the same, but the difference is that the assessor in the hospital has immediate back-up in the case of the child being seriously ill.

The preceding chapter has described the altered anatomy and physiology related to the child; in that chapter examples of applied anatomy and physiology have been provided. This chapter builds on some of those examples and places the assessment and monitoring of the child in context.

Assessment is a continuous, multistaged process and the foundation for decision-making, hence monitoring of the child's condition, will be determined by the data collected during the assessment phase. The nursing diagnosis phase is the analysis of data in order to identify patterns and create clear concise statements of the child/family's nursing problems. Nursing diagnosis helps to focus on the nursing problems and it differs from the medical model in that it offers a holistic approach (Aggleton and Chalmers, 2000). While debate exists over this fifth stage, it allows for reflection on the data gathered and then the child's and family's nursing needs can be appropriately identified and care planned.

This chapter will discuss what assessment is, the rationale for it, when it should be carried out and how it is carried out. An outline of how to assess a child's breathing, circulation and temperature will be discussed.

*Caring for Children and Families.* Edited by I. Peate and L. Whiting
© 2006 John Wiley & Sons Ltd

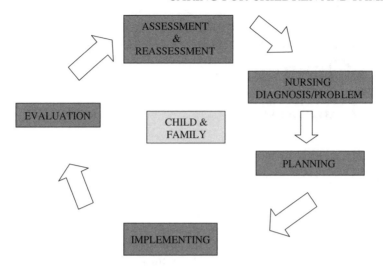

**Figure 7.1** The assessment cycle.

## WHAT IS FAMILY-CENTRED ASSESSMENT?

Assessment may be defined as:

> an activity which includes gathering data, interpreting the significance of the data, and deciding whether there is a need for further action. (Glasper and Campbell, 1995, p. 127)

Nursing models and philosophies can be incorporated into this stage of the nursing process to guide and structure the approach taken. The philosophy of family-centred care and partnership (Casey, 1988) should inform the whole nursing process in children's nursing. Parents may well be the experts at meeting many of their child's needs, thus recognition of this at the assessment phase is important before beginning to plan care. This challenges the entrenched views of the children's nurse, but for a family-centred approach to be developed this acknowledgement is essential (Smith *et al.*, 2001).

Assessment is a two-way process; information is exchanged and an opportunity is provided to develop a therapeutic relationship, with the nurse explaining why it is valuable to have an in-depth knowledge of the child and family. Information should be obtained from the child depending on their age, cognition and ability during the assessment process. Questioning and discussion should reflect their understanding. This approach ensures needs are assessed in partnership with the child and family.

The result of the assessment can be expressed in a nursing problem. Discussion of data generated from the nursing assessment with members of the multidisciplinary team leads to a holistic approach in meeting the child's and family's needs. Nursing care may then be planned with the child and family, implemented and evaluated for its effectiveness and reassessed continually for success.

## WHY ASSESS?

The aim of assessment is to provide an accurate picture of the patient's current problems (Crow *et al.*, 1995). Part of the skill of being a nurse is recognising when to assess, what to assess and knowing how to assess. Clinical judgements are made as a result of the nursing assessment.

Other important rationales for assessing are as follows.

- A child's condition can deteriorate rapidly and without warning; assessment and monitoring can alert the nurse to subtle changes, both physical and emotional, which can then be acted upon.
- Children may not be able to communicate how they are feeling or what their needs are.
- Assessment should facilitate individualised care for each and every child that is appropriate to their needs.
- It should acknowledge the family's need for support.
- It should identify problems that are not immediately obvious and that are not connected to the child's primary health need.

## WHEN TO ASSESS

Assessment is an ongoing process. It should be comprehensive and systematic, taking into account the physical, psychological, social and spiritual needs of the patients, clients and community (Nursing and Midwifery Council (NMC), 2004).

Assessment should be performed when:

- the child is first met. This can be in the accident and emergency department, the ward on admission or in outpatient/pre-admission clinics. It may be in the child's home or school environment.
- on the ward on a daily basis, to ascertain the relevance of the child's current plan of care and to identify the effectiveness of the care being delivered. Best practice suggests that assessment should be carried out at the commencement of each shift and when going into the child's home or school.
- the child's condition suddenly deteriorates with no warning. This may take the form of a rapid assessment in the case of a sudden collapse, and basic life-support guidelines will have to be instigated.
- a child with long-term health needs requires joint assessment in the form of a multidisciplinary team approach. This may be undertaken prior to discharge to enable seamless care and transition to the community environment.

## HOW TO ASSESS

Assessment may be formal and structured, as in cardiopulmonary assessment when a child is acutely ill, or it can use a recognised framework method of data collection, such as Roper *et al.* (1996). Assessment may be informal, such as the subconscious observations that the experienced practitioner tends to make when communicating with a child or family or when observing them from a distance.

It is essential that the child is included as long as their developmental age allows. Establish a rapport with them as soon as possible as this will assist in developing a sense of trust and help to gain the child's cooperation. This may not always be immediately possible, for example the child who may have life-threatening physical needs that must be addressed.

Data are generally gathered from three sources during the assessment process. Gaining data and facilitating a partnership in care requires three different skills (Casey, 1995):

1. observation
2. measurement
3. interview.

From these data, a picture of the child's and family's needs may be identified. These include both physical and psychosocial perspectives as well as their perceptions of their needs and concerns at that point in time.

### OBSERVATION

This process starts immediately before communication begins with the child and family. Making judgements about the child and noting their colour, positioning, behaviour, verbalisations and interactions with their family and environment may be done from across the room by using your sight and hearing. This will cause no distress or agitation to the child. Once sitting with the child and family, closer observation can occur. Redefinition of initial decisions at this point may occur. Alternatively, initial visual observations may alert you to this child's urgent needs for medical treatment before further needs can be assessed.

### MEASUREMENT

Many of the data that are collected through measurement will be directly related to the child's primary medical health needs. A measurement of vital signs and other physical parameters on admission will provide a baseline assessment of the child's condition. All children will need to have primary vital signs measured on admission; these may include temperature, pulse, blood pressure, respiratory rate and pain level. Weight must be recorded as medication and fluids will be calculated according to this. The need for other obser-

**Table 7.1** Some aspects of physical assessment that may be undertaken during the assessment stage

| | |
|---|---|
| weight | oxygen saturation levels |
| length (children under the age of 2 years, important for monitoring physical development) | peak expiratory flow rate (over 5 years of age, to measure tidal volume) |
| height | Glasgow coma scale (e.g. head injuries, unconscious child, some poisonings) |
| body mass index (children who have metabolic disorders or malnutrition) | neurovascular assessment (e.g. in the case of limb trauma or fractures) |
| head circumference | examination of skin for lesions/wound/ rashes/bruising |
| abdominal girth | |
| heart rate apex, radial and brachial pulses | urine analysis (performed on admission to detect abnormalities) |
| blood pressure | |
| respiratory rate: noting rate, depth and observation of work of breathing (use of accessory muscles, noises, chest expansion, colour) | blood glucose (known and suspected diabetic type 1 and 2 sufferers, alcohol overdose) |
| temperature | limb and joint movements (when injury has occurred or child complains of limb/joint pain) |
| fluid balance | |
| pain (use a recognised pain assessment chart; this is often referred to as the 'fifth vital sign') | |

vations to be measured will be determined by what the child's primary medical need is and how ill they are. This will usually be indicated in the medical notes. (See Table 7.1 for what this physical assessment may include.)

INTERVIEWING

The child and family are the primary source of verbal data during assessment. By asking open and closed questions, it should be possible to ascertain all the necessary information required in order to formulate a plan of nursing care. Consideration of the child's developmental stage is vital. As new information becomes available, this will have to be incorporated into your plan of care. When performing the initial assessment interview, the nurse should follow the guidelines below.

• Introduce himself or herself and identify the names of the family members present. Identify how the family wish to be addressed and record this on the assessment sheet. Identify who has parental responsibility at this point in time as it is not always the parents who accompany the child to the hospital.
• Attend to any urgent physical needs that the child may have, for example if the child is in pain, administer analgesia prior to completing the full assessment as both child and parent will be much more cooperative and willing participants if their physical needs are met.
• Outline the process of what your role is and how you will contribute to the child's care. Clarify the purpose of assessment as the child and family may

already have given their details to a range of other healthcare profession-als and can often be frustrated by having to answer more questions. There may be inconsistencies in the history which will not be recognised if an accu-rate assessment is not performed.

- Begin the interview with general questions such as asking the family to confirm their personal details, how they have been since their last admis-sion if a regular patient or how they have been at home prior to this admis-sion. This will also give you an idea as to the quality of historians the child and family are likely to be, and you may need to revise your later questions if you are requiring only minimal information. The parents may be very anxious and distressed, and this should be taken into account during the assessment interview.
- If possible, conduct the assessment in a private area with access to play materials for the child. Assure the family of the confidential nature of infor-mation and who will have access to it. The need to share information with regard to child-protection issues must occur and the family needs to be aware of this.
- If the child's and family's first language is not English, arrange for a suit-able interpreter at the earliest possible opportunity, if needed.
- Document carefully your assessment in the child's notes immediately and allow time for the child and parents to question and seek clarity regarding any aspects of hospitalisation or treatment planned.
- Be professional and calm: admission to hospital or having an unwell child is a huge distress for both the child and the family and first impressions are important.

## TOOLS FOR ASSESSMENT

The tools that are used for assessment must be reliable and valid and can take many forms, alerting the carer to the actual or potential problems of the child. Many of the tools utilised today are part of risk management, risk to the child (such as tissue viability risk) assessment and moving and handling risk assess-ment. Other well-recognised tools include pain-assessment tools and the Glasgow coma scale.

## TOOLS FOR RAPID ASSESSMENT

Assessment can be done as an urgent process in emergency situations. This will follow the basic life-support ABC algorithm (Resuscitation Council, 2000) of:

- **A**irway
- **B**reathing
- **C**irculation.

Problems identified are dealt with as they are found and care implemented immediately with ongoing evaluation of the child's condition by continuous reassessment and monitoring.

A rapid assessment of responsiveness may be performed by using the AVPU mnemonic (Advanced Life Support Group (ALSG), 2003). This is for very sick children and for use by experienced practitioners.

- **A**lert
- **V**oice-respond to voice
- **P**ain-response to pain
- **U**nconscious.

## TOOLS FOR CONTINUOUS ASSESSMENT

These can take many forms and some that are in general use are listed below in Table 7.2.

**Table 7.2** Some tools that may be used to assess the child

| Tool | Indications for use |
|---|---|
| Oral risk indicator tool | To identity the risk and extent of oral stomatitis, thus the need for mouth care to be included in the child's care plan. May be used for children who have received chemotherapy. |
| Tissue viability risk assessment | For identifying the risk of pressure ulcers. This may be used for a child who is unconscious, has special needs or a child on bed rest. |
| Moving and handling risk assessment | For identifying the potential moving and handling problems and the extent of the risk to child, family and staff. The occurrence of risk should also be assessed. Every infant, child and young person should have one completed on admission. |
| Pain-assessment tools (e.g. Wong, Baker faces) | A systematic method of identifying pain intensity and the evaluation of care given to alleviate pain. All children should have their pain level assessed on admission and as indicated. |
| Lund Bowder assessment chart for burns | This is used for children who have received burns to calculate the percentage of body surface area affected. |
| Croup score | The child who is admitted with croup can have the severity of their croup measured using a croup score, this measures degree of stridor and respiratory rate. |
| Glasgow coma scale | Should be used for all children when head trauma has occurred or if there is any concern about their level of consciousness. A modified version should be used for children under 4 years of age. |

## SYSTEMATIC ASSESSMENT

This involves the use of a model of nursing to guide the assessment process. Models of nursing are a means to provide detailed guidance, for the steps that need to be undertaken when planning and delivering nursing care (Aggleton and Chalmers, 2000).

Some models of nursing that may be used in child healthcare practice are:

- Casey's (1988) Family Centred Care Model
- Roper *et al.*'s (1996) Activities of Living Model
- Nottingham Model (Smith, 1995)
- Orem's Self Care Model (1970).

## ASSESSMENT IN PRACTICE

This section will concentrate on the assessment of breathing, circulation and body temperature monitoring as these are fundamental to the survival of all infants and children in the hospital or home setting regardless of whether their illness is mild or severe.

### BREATHING

**Introduction**

The accurate assessment of breathing and prompt treatment of any alterations identified is an essential skill for the children's nurse and cannot be empha- sised enough as disorders of the respiratory tract are one of the most common illnesses of childhood (ALSG, 2003). Any assessment of the respiratory status gives vital clues about the child's condition and must be performed rapidly, thoroughly and continuously. Disorders of breathing still carry a high mortal- ity rate in the UK (ALSG, 2003). Normal breathing should be effortless, and humans are generally not conscious of the act of breathing until it becomes abnormal (Roper *et al.*, 2000).

This section will address the role of the nurse in the assessment of breath- ing. Breathing is complex, and the health professional needs to understand the related anatomical and physiological principles fully in order to be able to administer nursing care; so referral to other texts and Chapter 6 is essential.

**Assessment**

Respiratory assessment involves interviewing, history-taking, physical exami- nation, observation, listening, auscultation and documentation. Equipment relating to respiratory function may also be used, for example an oxygen sat- uration monitor or an apnoea alarm. Recording respiratory rate is important

**Table 7.3** Normal respiratory rates for infants and children *(Source: MacGregor, 2000)*

| Child's age | Respiratory rate (breaths per minute) |
| --- | --- |
| newborn | 30–50 |
| 1 year | 26–40 |
| 2 years | 20–30 |
| 4 years | 20–30 |
| 6 years | 20–26 |
| 8 years | 18–24 |
| 10 years | 18–24 |
| adult | 12–20 |

as it forms a baseline against which the child's condition can be compared to in order to recognise improvement and deterioration. It is necessary for the monitoring of the child with respiratory distress, aids diagnosis and evaluates the child's response to medication that affects the respiratory system.

**Measuring respiratory rate**

A wealth of information may be gleaned by simply observing the child's respiratory pattern, and, as this is non-invasive, no added distress to the child should result. This should be done by observing the child and counting the rate of breathing for one full minute, timed by using a watch with a second hand. By observing the child or infant, the rate, depth, rhythm and movement of the chest wall can be identified. By listening, sounds associated with the noise of breathing such as wheeze, grunting or stridors and whether this occurs on inspiration or expiration can be determined.

As with any assessment, any deviation from 'normal' needs to be identified and you need to know the normal rate and type of respirations in relation to the child's age. The normal rates of respirations are presented in Table 7.3.

**Procedure for monitoring respirations**

Respiratory rate is the number of times a person inhales and exhales in one minute.

• Explain the procedure to the child and family. By taking the child's pulse rate first, you may begin to count the respiratory rate unknown to the child. This will enable you to perform a more accurate assessment of the child's respiratory rate as the older child may enhance the process of breathing.

• Using a watch with a second hand, observe the movement of the chest wall in the child for *one full minute*. For the infant, observe the rise and fall of their abdomen for *one full minute* as their respiratory pattern may not yet be regular and the use of their diaphragm is more apparent. Do not be tempted to measure for less than one full minute as abnormalities in the pattern of breathing may not be detected.

- Observe the depth of respiration. The depth of breathing is also known as the 'tidal volume' (Blow, 2001), that is the amount of air being moved in and out of the lungs in one minute. This will relate to the age of the child.
- Observe the rhythm of the infant's or child's breathing, e.g. is it regular or irregular?
- Document the findings in the child's observation chart and promptly report to senior nursing staff and/or medical staff any abnormalities, adjusting the child's care plan accordingly to meet their care needs.

This skill may be difficult initially, but with supervised practice and the support of a mentor/clinical facilitator will develop and confidence will grow. However, this is only part of the assessment and is insufficient to detect the child who may be in respiratory distress. The adequacy of breathing needs to be assessed. A rapid assessment needs to take place in the severely ill child, following the ABC (airway, breathing, circulation) approach (Resuscitation Council Guidelines, 2000); so knowledge of paediatric basic life support is required for this. It is useful to note that a child who is crying or talking will always have a patent airway, but a full respiratory assessment must be undertaken as the child's condition can deteriorate at any time and this will serve as a useful baseline.

For the child who is in respiratory distress and thereby not exhibiting a normal respiratory rate or pattern, you need to consider the following:

- work of breathing
- effectiveness of breathing
- effects of inadequate respirations (ALSG, 2003).

---

**Activity**
*James is a 6-year-old who has been admitted to your ward with an exacerbation of his asthma. Outline how you would assess his respiratory status.*

---

You may have considered some of the following procedures.

- Check patency of airway: assess his breathing by noting his respiratory rate, depth of breathing and rhythm and note whether or not he is using his abdominal muscles.
- Then assess the work of breathing by looking at his chest to see what muscles he is using. He may have intercostal or subcostal recession; note if he has a tracheal tug or if he is using his neck muscles.
- Check James's pulse rate and note the degree of tachycardia.
- Observe James's nostrils – they may be flaring.
- See if James can speak: if he is in severe respiratory distress, he may not be able to speak.

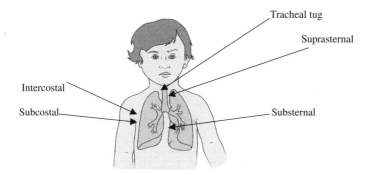

**Figure 7.2** Location of recession when the work of breathing is altered.

- Listen for noises. James will probably have a wheeze, but an absence of a wheeze may present with severe obstruction of his airways.
- Note the position James is sitting in; he may be sitting and leaning forward.
- Note James's skin colour: is he pink, pale or cyanosed? Cyanosis is a late sign and indicative of respiratory arrest.
- Assess James's level of consciousness: is he alert, drowsy, irritable, agitated, anxious, responsive to pain or unconscious? James should have his oxygen saturation levels checked.
- If James knows how to do a peak flow, record one.

**Work of breathing**

As part of the physical assessment, the work of breathing is assessed.

*Recession*

This is an in-drawing of the soft tissues over the chest wall and it is described depending on the area involved (see Figure 7.2).

Recession indicates an increase in respiratory effort and respiratory distress. It can be described as mild, moderate or severe depending on the depth, and this relies on clinical experience and judgement. You may notice that James has intercostal and subcostal recession on arrival by looking at his chest. This must be reported to senior staff immediately. If his condition deteriorates, he may develop substernal recession and a tracheal tug as the work of breathing increases. If James is obese, the presence of intercostal and subcostal recession may not be so obvious and this needs to be considered.

**Respiratory sounds**

Normal breathing is quiet and there is no sound heard. While counting the respiratory rate, the nurse must be alert to any sounds heard, whether they are on inspiration or expiration, and be able to interpret their meaning.

*Wheezing*

Wheeze can occur on inspiration or expiration and is characterised by a whistling sound that is caused by the forcing of air through narrow airways that is most often associated with an exacerbation of asthma and bronchiolitis. An inspiratory wheeze is indicative of upper airway obstruction, for example croup or presence of a foreign body, an expiratory wheeze is indicative of lower airway obstruction, for example bronchiolitis or asthma. Recession may accompany wheezing. Williams and Asquith (2000) advise that in a child with a loss of a wheeze who has been previously wheezy very little air movement may be taking place, indicating the onset of respiratory failure. Thus, the audibility of the wheeze must be considered in light of vital signs and other physical signs and not taken as a reliable indicator of the child's condition. James is quite likely to have a wheeze as he appears to be having a moderate exacerbation of his asthma. If his condition deteriorates, this wheeze may disappear and his chest would become silent, which is a life-threatening sign. An absence of a wheeze may represent a severe obstruction and, with improvement, wheezing may become more prominent (Barnes, 2003).

*Stridor*

This is a harsh sound produced by air being forced through oedematous airways. It can be on inspiration indicating oedema above the epiglottis, as in croup and epiglottitis; it may also be accompanied by recession. An inspiratory and expiratory stridor may indicate the child has an abnormality below the level of the vocal cords. Stridor in the child indicates acute respiratory illness. The degree of stridor may be exacerbated by distressing the child; so this should be avoided at all costs. Stridor may also be present in a child who has inhaled a foreign body, as the foreign body moves, the stridor may intensify or decrease (Dhillon and East, 1994).

*Grunting*

Grunting is heard in infants who have respiratory distress. The infant is exhaling against a partially closed glottis in an attempt to maintain the functional residual capacity of the alveoli. This is an indication of respiratory distress.

**Use of accessory muscles**

*Head bobbing*

This sign will only be seen in infants and is indicative of respiratory distress. The infant uses the scalene and sternomastoid muscle as an accessory muscle when the work of breathing is increased (Wong *et al.*, 2003). This causes the head to bob up and down with each breath, thus making breathing ineffectual. While James will not be head bobbing, he may well be using his neck muscles if his exacerbation of asthma becomes severe (Thorax, 2003). This requires immediate reporting to senior nursing staff and/or doctors.

### Nasal flaring

By looking at the infant or child's nostrils, it is possible to see them flaring when the work of breathing is increased. By enlarging the nostrils, the child is attempting to maintain a patent airway and reduce nasal resistance. It may be intermittent or continuous and should be reported as either minimal or marked. It is especially seen in infants who are in respiratory distress. James may have nasal flaring, and you need to record and report this.

### Respiratory rate

As previously discussed, you will record James's respiratory rate for one full minute. If it is more than 30 breaths per minute, James's asthma could be said to be severe (Thorax, 2003). This needs to be considered and collated with his other vital signs: heart rate, oxygen saturation levels, his ability to speak and peak flow rate.

### Breathlessness

It is important to note if James is breathless and when this occurs. This may occur at rest, when walking or talking, when sleeping or on exertion, such as when running. In infants it is essential to note if they become breathless when feeding as it is a useful sign when assessing respiratory distress.

### Ability to speak

The child who presents with respiratory distress will do so in varying degrees ranging from moderate to life-threatening. Their ability to speak is an indication of the level of distress and should be noted as part of the assessment process. James has been admitted with a moderate exacerbation of his asthma and should be able to speak. However, if he presents with a severe exacerbation of asthma, he may well be too breathless to talk or may only manage single words. It is important to avoid asking the child questions directly in this instance and seek assistance from senior nursing staff. The child should either be nursed in a resuscitation room and have immediate access to a resuscitation trolley or, if in the home, an ambulance should be called.

**Effectiveness of breathing**

The effectiveness of breathing is determined by auscultation of the chest and this will be undertaken by an appropriately trained professional, indicating the amount of air being inspired and expired. Looking at the chest of children and the abdomen of infants will also assist in determining the effectiveness of breathing.

**Effects of inadequate respirations**

*Heart rate*

Inadequate respirations will have an adverse effect on heart rate as hypoxia leads to tachycardia. Consideration of the child's temperature, medication received and levels of distress may all contribute to a rise in their heart rate so this must be given due consideration when assessing the child's respiratory status, thus indicating the need for frequent if not continuous assessment. If James's heart rate is more than 120 beats per minute, he is in the severe exacerbation category (Thorax, 2003).

*Cyanosis or skin colour*

Colour changes in the skin range from mottling and pallor to cyanosis. In the mucous membranes, the lips, face, legs and arms, cyanosis (the presence of a bluish tinge) may be observed (ALSG, 2003). This is a very worrying sign and needs urgent treatment. This results from hypoxia due to poor gas exchange, decreased cardiac output and obstruction of the airway. These can all result from either acute or chronic conditions. Providing James has no underlying medical conditions, his colour should be normal on admission but may be pale because of his current condition. Any changes in James's colour needs prompt reporting.

*Psychological status*

In an infant or child who presents with respiratory distress, assessment of their psychological status is important. The child who is agitated or frightened may well be hypoxic. They may also be listless. Noting how the child responds to their parents, the environment and familiar objects can determine their state of alertness. If this cannot be ascertained, a more detailed examination is required of their neurological function. If it is suspected that the child has epiglottitis, it is essential that they are not distressed unnecessarily. When assessing James, it will be important to note his level of consciousness. This can be ascertained by noting his answers to questions that you would expect him to know the answers to and how he interacts with his environment and with treatment being administered.

**Other terms used in respiratory assessment**

These terms are terms that you may need to become familiar with.

*Apnoea*

Apnoea is the absence of breathing for 20 seconds or more, (MacGregor, 2000). There are many causes of apnoea ranging from respiratory, neurological, metabolic and obstruction (as in the case of enlarged tonsils and adenoids). It is recognised that pre-term infants (generally less than 32 weeks' gestation) have apnoeic episodes, and these can be effectively managed with stimulation and the administration of medication along with appropriate nursing care. The infant or child that presents with apnoea will need a detailed assessment and close monitoring.

*Cough*

The term 'cough' on its own is relatively meaningless. It must be considered in terms of its characteristics and with other symptoms (Lewis, 1999). A cough results from irritation of the cough receptors in the pharynx, larynx and bronchi (Tortora and Grabowski, 2003). A cough may be dry and non-productive, as in the case of asthma, or productive and producing sputum, as in the case of a child with cystic fibrosis or pneumonia. Young children tend to be unable to expectorate their sputum, swallowing it instead, which may lead to vomiting. It is always useful to ask the parents if they have noted any sputum in the vomitus.

It may be paroxysmal (uncontrollable) as in pertussis (whooping cough) or due to inhalation of a foreign body. There is a sudden onset of coughing spasms and these are forceful and multiple. In the case of pertussis, there is a characteristic whoop at the end of the coughing episode, but infants may not whoop and may still become apnoeic (Williams and Asquith, 2000).

The cough may be present at night only, which is termed 'nocturnal cough'. In the case of croup (laryngotracheobronchitis), the cough is a distinctive seal-like bark (ALSG, 2003) and referred to as a 'croupy cough'. A cough may become habitual and this must be considered when no organic cause can be identified.

The role of the nurse is to determine the presence, frequency, depth, sound of the cough and any associated trigger factors (Jenkins, 2003). The nurse also needs to support the child and family during the coughing phase, instigating treatment as prescribed to ensure the child's normal routines are returned to as soon as possible. When assessing a child, it will be important to ask about the presence of coughing and to identify any factors that trigger coughing. Note if the child is producing any sputum and what relieves the cough.

**Table 7.4** Position of saturation probes *(Source: Hockenberry* et al., *2005)*

| Age group | Probe position | Probe type |
|---|---|---|
| Infant | Across the palm of the hand, with the probe sited at the base of the little finger<br>On the outer aspect of the foot, with the probe sited at the base of the little toe<br>On the Achilles area | Self-adhesive probe |
| Young child | The finger or big toe<br>As above | Self-adhesive probe |
| Older child | Finger or toe<br>Ear lobe | Self-adhesive probe<br>Non-disposable clip probe<br>Finger probe |

**Monitoring respiratory status**

*Pulse oximetry*

Pulse oximetry is well recognised as a simple, useful, non-invasive method of recording oxygen saturation levels in arterial blood in infants and children (Van der Mosel, 1994). Pulse oximetry should be utilised for any infant or child that presents with respiratory distress of any degree. It is important that the user is educated and familiar with the equipment before using it even though they are now used routinely in patient care. A normal pulse saturation level is 95–98% in room air (Sims, 1996). Pulse oximetry can detect hypoxia before the infant or child has visible signs (Hanna, 1995), but must be used in conjunction with the nurse's clinical evaluation skills and is not a replacement for this. Heart rate is also recorded as blood flow is pulsatile.

When positioning an oxygen saturation probe on an infant or child, suggested places are identified in Table 7.4.

It is *always* advisable to refer to the manufacturer's instructions when using an oxygen saturation probe.

**Nursing care of an infant or child with pulse oximetry**

Consider Emma, who is 3 years of age and has attended the accident and emergency department with pyrexia, chest pain, productive cough and vomiting. She is likely to have a self-adhesive finger probe in place to monitor her oxygen saturation levels. You will have given Emma and her family a full explanation of this procedure before starting the monitoring and will have obtained their consent. When setting up the pulse oximetry monitor, you will have configured the lower and upper alarm limits for her oxygen saturation levels, and the low and high alarm for her heart rate and will have checked the audibility of the alarm. Setting the alarm limits should be discussed with the medical team as they need to be aware of possible deteriorations/improvements and the prescribing of appropriate treatment in the event of the child's condition altering. Emma's oxygen saturation level should be 92% or more in room air as her asthma is moderately exacerbated (Thorax, 2003), indicating that a lower alarm limit of 92% would be set in this case, thus demonstrating the need for close nursing and medical observation.

You will note the signal displayed on the monitor and the wave form being shown. This is important as it is indicative of the reliability of the reading. The probe site needs to be changed every two hours as it is possible for the child to receive burns to the area directly below the light source (Wong *et al.*, 2003). Changing the probe site must be documented and included as part of Emma's care plan. The probe should be secured according to the manufacturer's instructions only and with the equipment they have provided. Using tapes and bandages can lead to skin damage, pressure ulcers, burns and false recordings.

If Emma's saturation monitor alarms, respond to her promptly and look at her. Are her physical signs compatible with the reading on the monitor? If Emma's saturation level is dropping, seek assistance from a senior staff member. Her other vital signs also need to be considered so that a full and accurate assessment is being considered.

Emma may need to commence oxygen therapy if her saturation does drop and she is showing signs of increasing respiratory distress. The continuous monitoring of her saturation levels and the response to oxygen therapy, noting the amount of oxygen she is receiving, will need to be documented in her observation chart. If Emma's vital signs are within normal limits, the position of the probe needs to be considered, making sure that the probe is correctly positioned.

There are also limitations to the use of pulse oximetry and these must be considered (Table 7.5).

Other factors that may affect pulse oximetry readings are:

- incorrect probe size – must be suitable for the weight of the child
- nail varnish

**Table 7.5** Factors affecting pulse oximetry readings

- Pulse oximetry cannot differentiate between the different types of gas molecules as in carbon monoxide poisoning so will read as for oxyhaemoglobin (Carroll, 1993).
- Excessive movement will affect the sensor.
- If peripheral perfusion is poor, the readings may be inaccurate.
- It will not consider the child's haemoglobin level; therefore it cannot be relied upon to assess the oxygen carrying capacity of the blood (Van der Mosel, 1994)
- If the child is oedematous, inaccuracies are likely.
- Bright light from external sources and high intensity heat may affect readings.
- If intravenous dyes for investigations have been used, inaccurate saturation levels may result.

- dirty probe and dirty probe site (Wong *et al.*, 2003)
- incorrect sitting of probe – wrong way up
- low battery.

## Peak expiratory flow rate (PEFR) monitoring

Peak expiratory flow rate meters are used to measure pulmonary function in children with respiratory conditions such as asthma. PEFR measures the rate at which air is exhaled from the lungs and is measured in litres per second or minute. In order to know if the child is achieving a normal peak flow, their height must be recorded and this plotted against a normogram, which will identify their predicted peak flow. It should be used in all children with asthma or other respiratory conditions when they are 5 years of age or older. In the child with asthma, the peak flow meter is best if used frequently so that diaries can be maintained and treatment adjusted according to their self-management plan.

---

**Activity**
*Chloe is 5 and a half years and has not used a peak flow meter previously. You need to teach her and her parents how to use the peak flow meter. Think about how you would do this.*

---

You may have considered the following procedure.

1. Explain the procedure to Chloe and her parents and the reasons why it is used.
2. Place the measurement bar at zero.
3. Ask Chloe to stand up if not contraindicated.
4. Holding the peak flow meter horizontally, ask Chloe to take a deep breath in, then place the mouthpiece on her tongue and ask her to seal her lips and blow out as hard and fast as she can.
5. Read the number the measurement bar is indicating.
6. After resting and breathing normally for a few seconds, repeat steps 2–5 twice more.
7. Record the best reading and document.

If Chloe has her own mouthpiece, this should be cleaned according to manufacturer's instructions. Otherwise disposable mouthpieces should be used and disposed of after each use.

If the child records their peak flows regularly, the reading should be compared to their own baseline measurement. If Chloe had regularly recorded her peak flow and they were now less than 50% of her normal best or predicted value, this indicates that she is having a severe exacerbation of her asthma. If the peak flow reading is less than 33% of her best or predicted value, her asthma would be life threatening (Thorax, 2003). This indicates the importance of recording accurate peak flows in all children with asthma who are over 5 years of age.

To recap, respiratory assessment must be comprehensive and systematically performed. When assessing the child, the nurse needs to be aware of:

- normal parameters;
- respiratory rate – count for one full minute;
- the work of breathing – recession, use of accessory muscles, grunting in the infant, noise of breathing, flaring nostrils, breathlessness;
- the effectiveness of breathing – chest movement and air movement within the chest;
- the effect of breathing – heart rate, colour and mental status;
- oxygen saturation levels;
- presence of cough.

Careful assessment, continual monitoring, prompt reporting and treatment are essential as respiratory illness remains a major cause of childhood morbidity and mortality. Respiratory assessment as outlined here can be undertaken rapidly but requires the nurse to have a good understanding of paediatric anatomy and related physiology. Recognising the infant or child in respiratory distress and acting on those findings should prevent respiratory failure from occurring; therefore, this is a fundamental skill.

## BLOOD PRESSURE

Blood pressure is defined as the force of the blood against the walls of the vessels in which it is contained (Tortora and Grabowski, 2003). In order to understand the factors that affect blood pressure in infants and children, the student needs to be aware of related anatomy and physiology (Chapter 6). Blood pressure is reported as the systolic measurement over the diastolic measurement.

*Systolic pressure* is the maximum pressure of the blood against the walls of the vessels following ventricular contraction, and *diastolic pressure* is the minimum pressure of the blood against the walls of the vessels when the aortic valve is closing and the ventricles are relaxing (Mallet and Dougherty, 2000).

The two terms that you are likely to encounter in relation to abnormalities of blood pressure are *hypotension*, which means the systolic blood pressure is below the normal range. The main causes of this in children are septic, hypo-volaemic or cardiogenic shock. *Hypertension* is when the systolic reading is higher than the normal range. In the child this could be due to renal disease, some congenital heart defects, medication, pain, raised intracranial pressure or fluid overload. Measuring blood pressure gives vital clues about the health status of the child and, like any other vital sign, a single reading is of little value, and serial recordings are indicated when any abnormality is found.

You also need to be aware of the normal ranges of blood pressure (Table 7.6). Blood pressure is a less reliable vital sign in children than in adults as infants and children's cardiovascular systems compensate well and can maintain a normal blood pressure until shock is severe, thus systolic blood

**Table 7.6** 'Normal' blood pressure range for infants and children *(Source: MacGregor, 2000)*

| Age | Male (measured in mm Hg) | Female (measured in mm Hg) |
|---|---|---|
| Newborn | 70/55 | 65/55 |
| 5 years | 95/56 | 94/56 |
| 10 years | 100/62 | 102/62 |
| 15 years | 115/65 | 111/67 |
| Adult | 121/70 | 112/60 |

pressure readings may give a more reliable reading than diastolic ones (ALSG, 2003). Hypotension is a late and very worrying sign in a sick child and requires immediate medical management.

Blood pressure in children may be recorded manually, using a sphygmomanometer or, more commonly, an electronic device such as a Dinamap™. This equipment calculates the blood pressure by measuring the frequency of ultrasonic waves reflected by the movement of the surface of the blood vessels (Ball and Bindler, 2006), whereas the manual method measures the actual blood pressure at that point in time. While it is now being recommended that children have their blood pressure measured using the auscultatory method (Committee on Blood Pressure Monitoring in Clinical Practice, 2004), competence in both of these non-invasive procedures is required in the student.

### When to take a child's blood pressure

Recording a child's blood pressure can often be challenging, yet there are many reasons why it is necessary to record blood pressure.

- It provides a baseline of the child's condition on admission.
- It aids in assessing the child's cardiovascular system.
- It may be used to monitor the effect of medication (e.g. anti-hypertension medication).
- It may assist in the diagnosis of disease, e.g. cardiac disease, renal disease.
- It monitors variations in a child's condition.
- It may identify an additional health need that is not immediately obvious (e.g. undiagnosed renal disease or a neurological defect).

### Procedure for recording a child's blood pressure

One of the most important components in recording an infant's or child's blood pressure is choosing the correct cuff size – whether their blood pressure is being recorded manually or electronically. The normal site for measuring a child's blood pressure is the upper limbs. The child's legs may be used, but this should be documented clearly in the child's observation chart. The gold standard is manual recording, and the same principle of correct cuff sizing is required.

To select the correct cuff size, compare the cuff with the size of the child's upper arm. The bladder of the cuff should cover at least 80 % of the circumference of the limb being used (Beevers *et al.*, 2001). The bladder width should cover two-thirds of the upper arm or thigh, depending on which is being used. If the bladder is too small, the reading will be falsely high; if it is too large, the pressure will be a falsely low.

When undertaking serial recordings of blood pressure, the aim should be to undertake them under the same circumstances, that is if the child is sitting, lying or standing and at a similar time of day. This should be noted and considered. Providing education to ensure safe handling during use and in the event of a mercury spillage has been undertaken, mercury sphygmomanometers may still be used (Medical Devices Agency, 2000), but, if they exist, alternatives are preferable.

## To measure blood pressure manually

- Select the correct cuff size and wrap it snugly round the child's arm having already explained the procedure to the child and elicited their cooperation. The arm should be supported by pillows and at heart level.
- Try to take the reading when the child has been resting or is sitting calmly. If the child is upset, it is probably not the best time to take their blood pressure. Loosen any tight clothing on the upper arm/limb. Right or left arms may be used.
- Palpate for the brachial pulse and place the stethoscope over the pulse area, checking that the diaphragm of the stethoscope is placed over the artery with it switched to the diaphragm. In those under 5 years of age, a Doppler is preferable to a stethoscope to audibly hear the brachial pulse. Making sure the air-escape valve is closed, pump the cuff up until the gauge rises and no beat can be auscualted. Continue until the gauge rises to another 30 mmHg over the estimated systolic pressure (Beevers *et al.*, 2001).
- Your eye level needs to be in line with that of the top of the fluid level in the sphygmomanometer; otherwise, errors may occur. Concentration is essential as skill is required to hear phasing of Korotkoff's sounds. Korotkoff's sounds are caused by the blood flowing through the brachial artery during the peak of each systole and become louder as the cuff pressure is released. The first sound will be a sharp thud as the pressure on the cuff is released and this is the systolic reading. As the artery is no longer constricted, blood flows freely and the sounds become muffled at first and then disappear, thus giving the diastolic reading. Both of these values should be noted.

- Slowly release the valve at a rate of 2–3 mmHg per second while watching the gauge.
- Note the number at which the first return of pulse is heard (Korotkoff's sounds), this is the systolic pressure.
- Continue to release the air valve. The National High Blood Pressure Education Programme Working Group (2004) suggests that the disappearance of sounds, Korotkoff 5, should be used as the diastolic unless sounds continue to 0 mmHg. If this occurs, Korotkoff 4, a muffling of sound, should be used as the diastolic. Korotkoff's sounds are not reliably heard in all children under the age of 1 year and in those less than 5 years of age, thus indicating the needs for oscillometry and Dopplers to be used (MacGregor, 2000).
- Remove cuff and record results as per local policy in child's records, reporting any deviations from normal range. The blood pressure needs to be recorded to the nearest 2 mmHg to maintain accuracy and should not be rounded off.

### Recording blood pressure using electronic blood pressure monitor

- Having explained the procedure to the child and family and gained their cooperation, place the correctly sized cuff around the child's arm, ensuring their arm is supported at heart level and their comfort.
- Activate the equipment according to the manufacturer's recommendations, ensuring that you are familiar with those recommendations.
- It may be necessary to distract the child as the equipment is often adversely affected by the movement of the child, thus causing the cuff to re-tighten and start again, distressing the child further and then often not providing a reading.
- Note the readings and document them once you have removed the cuff from the child's arm.

The frequency of monitoring a child's blood pressure is dependent on their clinical condition. If there is doubt over any of the readings, the need for several measurements may be indicated.

## BODY TEMPERATURE RECORDING

Often the first indication that a child is unwell will present itself as an increase in their body temperature. The accurate recording of body temperature is an important aspect of clinical assessment. Maintaining a normal body temperature is essential for normal growth and development (Bee and Boyd, 2004).

### What is body temperature recording?

One reason for an increase in body temperature is a result of complex interactions between exogenous pyrogens, such as bacteria or viruses, invading the body cells triggering the release of endogenous pyrogens. The pyrogens then travel in the blood to the hypothalamus and either directly or by creating prostaglandins alter the 'normal set point'. As the blood flowing through the hypothalamus will be considered to be lower than the new set point, the body's response will be heat conservation, and mechanisms to do this are then initiated (MacGregor, 2000). Other reasons are hypothalamic disturbances or post-cardiac surgery.

Children are also at risk of becoming hypothermic quickly when injured or ill, and this must also be given consideration. A normal core body temperature for a newborn infant will be between 36.5 °C and 37.6 °C (Hockenberry *et al.*, 2005). As the child grows, the normal body temperature reflects a decreasing basic metabolic rate, and for an older child a range of 36 °C to 37.5 °C may be considered to be within normal parameters and this will vary depending on the site measured. An axillary measurement may be 1 °C less than an oral measurement, and a rectal measurement 1 °C more. This is an important consideration when documenting temperature measurements and the site used should be noted.

---

**Activity**
*An 8-year-old boy called Mital is brought to the medical room at school by his teacher who says that Mital was feeling hot earlier but has now started to shiver. How will you assess Mital? You should follow some of the procedures below.*

---

**Measuring body temperature**

Temperature in healthy and ill children can be measured by various routes: tympanically, orally, axillary, peripherally or rectally. The rectal route is still used but not routinely and should be avoided. It should only be used if no other route is possible or the child's clinical condition dictates this method. The potential for perforation of the rectum is high, and measuring temperature in this way is highly intrusive.

In the newborn, the axilla or peripheral routes are more desirable routes to use to record body temperature. There are a variety of thermometers available for clinical use, and familiarity for accurate use is essential. These include infrared tympanic devices, single-use disposable thermometers (ideal for use in children with confirmed or suspected infectious diseases). The choice of thermometer will depend on the child's condition, their developmental stage and what is available. Glass mercury thermometers should not be used except in the case of the hypothermic child where rectal monitoring is advocated (ALSG, 2003). Rectal measurements will not be discussed in this chapter.

As part of assessing the child's temperature, their appearance should also be noted as the child with an increase in their body temperature will often have a flushed face, low energy levels, malaise and an increased respiratory

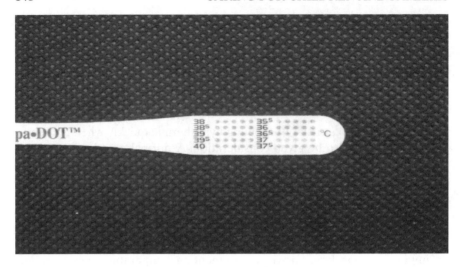

**Figure 7.3** A disposable thermometer.

rate and heart rate. A child's heart rate will increase by 10 beats per minute for each 0.5 °C rise in temperature above their core temperature (Barnes, 2003). When measuring body temperature, the child's general condition should be noted. Figure 7.3 demonstrates a disposable thermometer.

**Tympanic route**

This method records the temperature of the tympanic membrane as it is considered that the tympanic temperature closely reflects that of the core body temperature due to the proximity of the tympanic membrane to the hypothalamus and the fact that it shares a blood supply (Rogers, 1991). It uses an infrared light to record the temperature.

The tympanic route is a fast, convenient method of measuring temperature. An infrared light detects thermal radiation providing a rapid reading, hence why this method is so popular. Accurate measurement depends upon correct technique. This route should not be used in children with suspected or known ear infections or those who have had recent ear surgery. The presence of ear wax in the canal will provide an inaccurate reading. The same ear should be utilised when recording the temperature frequently and the child needs to be in the same ambient temperature for 20 minutes to provide greater accuracy (Childs *et al.*, 1999).

1. Gather equipment, tympanic thermometer and disposable probe cover.
2. Wash hands.
3. Explain procedure to the child and family and gain their cooperation.

4. Position child on parent's lap or on bed/chair if old enough to cooperate.
5. With a young child, stabilise their head, while in the supine position, and turn their head so the ear is uppermost for ease of access.
6. *For a child under 1 year of age*: gently pull the pinna of the ear straight back and down. Approach the ear from behind to direct the tip of the probe anteriorly, thus making sure that the tip of the thermometer is aimed at the tympanic membrane. This method is not suitable for young babies as the probe is generally too large for the size of their ear canals.
7. Gently place the probe in the ear canal as far as possible, ensuring a good seal and turn on scanner.
8. When measurement is completed, remove probe, note reading and record in child's observation chart.
9. Dispose of probe cover, wash hands.
10. *For the child more than 1 year of age*: gently pull the pinna up and back and follow steps 7–9.

There has been a lot of research undertaken on the effectiveness of tympanic temperature recordings with variable findings as to the effectiveness of such a method. Try to locate some of this research and formulate your views about the accuracy of this method of temperature taking.

**Axillary measurements**

The axillary route is often used for measuring temperature in the newborn, children with special needs, the unconscious child and those with any structural abnormalities that preclude alternative routes, and this is usually the route of choice. Electronic thermometers, digital or disposable single-use thermometers are used for measuring temperature via this route. The disadvantage to using this route is that readings may not be as accurate as other methods as the length of time it takes for some devices to measure (up to three minutes with a disposable thermometer) can be challenging for the child to remain in the required position for that length of time.

1. Having explained the procedure to the child and gained their cooperation, wash hands.
2. Loosen child's clothing.
3. Place thermometer in its protective sheath if electronic and position in the axilla, ensuring that the axilla is dry and that good skin contact occurs. If using a disposable thermometer, such as a TEMPA dot™, ensure the dots are against the child's torso.
4. Ask the child to hold their arm either by their side or across their chest for the required amount of time. If using an electronic device, this will create an audible sound when the temperature is recorded. If it is a disposable thermometer, this must be left *in situ* for the required length of time as per manufacturer's instructions.

5. Remove the probe/disposable thermometer after the required time according to manufacturer's instructions. An electronic thermometer will have an audible tone indicating it has measured temperature.
6. When measurement is completed, remove probe, note reading and record in child's observation chart.
7. Dispose of probe cover and wash hands.

**Oral measurement**

This route is generally only used in the older child as there is always a risk of the younger child biting the thermometer and being unable to cooperate by holding the thermometer with their mouth closed. Oral temperature measurement should only be used with cooperative, alert children for safety reasons.

1. Having explained the procedure to the child and gained their cooperation, wash hands.
2. Place the oral probe covered with a disposable sheath or disposable thermometer under the child's tongue, in the sublingual pocket.
3. Ask the child to close their mouth.
4. Following manufacturer's recommendations, remove on hearing audible tone or after required time length if using disposable device.
5. Read and record temperature.
6. Dispose of waste and wash hands.

As with any other vital-sign measurement, a single temperature reading is of little value, and serial recordings will identify a trend associated with the child's temperature. Temperature measurement needs to be accurate as treatment may be instigated on the findings and inaccurate measurements may lead to inaccurate treatment. If the child feels hotter or cooler than the measurement recorded, re-measure using a different device and a different route is advocated. Environmental factors need to be considered when recording a temperature. If a child has had a hot or cold drink, they should not have their temperature recorded orally; similarly, if they have just had a shower/bath, the axilla route should be avoided.

## BLOOD GLUCOSE MEASUREMENT AND MONITORING

As part of a newborn's or child's assessment and ongoing care, blood glucose measurement and monitoring is required for a number of reasons. The child may be susceptible to hypoglycaemia, be unconscious, on steroid treatment or more commonly have type 1 diabetes mellitus. Capillary blood is generally used to measure the glucose level.

Blood glucose monitoring is an essential skill and one that should only be undertaken by trained personnel as familiarity with finger/heel pricking devices and technique is required, as is an ability to use blood glucose strips and measuring devices, along with possessing the knowledge of how to interpret the results and the ability to liaise with other professional colleagues.

## MONITORING THE SICK CHILD

Monitoring the sick child is now commonplace on the children's ward and occasionally even in the home environment in the case of an oxygen-dependent infant or child by non-invasive means. Monitoring is the repetitive or continuous activity of making observation and measurements of a patient and adjusting the treatment plan accordingly while measuring the effectiveness of those treatment interventions. Monitoring can also be diagnostic and can save lives. The patient must always remain the priority and monitoring must not distract the nurse's attention away from the patient. It may involve electronic equipment but can equally involve other tools such as a pain-assessment tool.

The purpose of monitoring is to guide the management of that particular patient at that time. It may be continuous or intermittent. The nurse needs to be able to accurately interpret the data that are being displayed and be aware of the factors that may affect their validity, for example if the child is on continuous cardiac monitoring, you need to be able to identify and interpret the tracings.

The goal of monitoring (Williams and Asquith, 2000) should be:

- to evaluate the physiological status of the child and follow the course of acute illness or chronic illness in the case of a child at home;
- directed towards the physiological alterations that are pertinent to the child's altered physiology at the time;
- to assess the adequacy of vital organ function;
- to evaluate the results of pharmacological and physiological interventions;
- to monitor the therapeutic and toxic effects of certain drugs;
- to aid the early detection of complications by providing alarms that identify significant changes in the child's condition;
- to provide a permanent record of the child's physiological status;
- to assess the child's discomfort and the effects of methods to relieve that discomfort as in patient-controlled analgesia;
- to determine the need for other interventions such as artificial airway and breathing support;
- safe and do the child no harm.

It is the status of the child's condition that will indicate the need for monitoring, thus the need for an individual, holistic approach. As practitioners, the need to be aware of the benefits and pitfalls of using technology in practice while ensuring the best outcome for the children that access our services is paramount.

> **Activity:**
> *Identify the type of monitoring devices that are available in your area. Do you know what they monitor and how to interpret the data? Identify the negative aspects of using monitors.*

## DOCUMENTING VITAL SIGNS

Recording vital signs is a skill to be developed, as is documentation. It is an integral component of nursing practice. Little written material exists about how to document observations, with many variations in practice and in the type of observations that are available. In clinical practice the premise is that if it is not documented then it has not been done.

Recording vital signs is part of the professional duty of care owed to the patient. Any failure to maintain a reasonable standard of patient records could be professional misconduct and may be subjected to professional conduct proceedings. Contemporary records should be maintained with vital signs documented on the correct chart as soon as possible with written evaluation to record actions taken documented clearly in the child's nursing/medical records, for example a doctor needed to be called as the child was found to have a tachycardia. Documentation of vital signs should follow local policy and this should be in accordance with NMC (2002). This also involves interpreting the vital signs as they are documented and comparing them with those recorded previously to identify trends, improvements, deteriorations and response to treatments.

When documenting vital signs, it is best to do this on a graph chart, with the readings represented as a dot rather than a numerical recording. The dots should be joined in a straight line rather than a curve, as deteriorations in a child's condition using this method are more easily identifiable. There should be a separate section for each recording: temperature, pulse, blood pressure and respiratory rate, so that as each measurement can be recorded clearly and viewed at a glance in order that patterns and trends are identified quickly. This is the only sure method of identifying a child's deteriorating condition, improvement in their clinical status and trends in response to their treatment.

## CONCLUSION

This chapter, closely related to the preceding chapter, has identified the importance of assessment and what it is and the purpose of monitoring. The procedure and skills required for undertaking the fundamentals of any assessment on any child have been discussed along with the need for serial measurements and accurate documentation identified. Knowledge of age-appropriate vital signs and equipment is essential if assessment is to be accurate. The general appearance of the child is a paramount indicator of their condition. Remember the family: the child is not the only one being assessed and treated; the family will provide invaluable information and assistance in assessing the child.

While there has been much research undertaken on temperature and blood pressure measurement in children, practice still demonstrates many variations with patient preference often being cited as the rationale for undertaking certain procedures. While patient preference is important, accuracy should always be the aim when undertaking any patient assessment. Pain is often recognised as the fifth vital sign and this must not be omitted on assessment; it has not been discussed in this chapter.

The skills required for assessing the child in the hospital or in the community setting are identical but contingency plans for those working in the community need to be in place on identification of the sick child in the school, home or clinic. The boundaries between home and hospital must remain clear with the home providing a place of sanctuary for the child and family as much as possible.

# REFERENCES

Advanced Life Support Group (ALSG) (2003) *Advanced Paediatric Life Support: The practical approach* (4th edn). London: BMJ Publishing Group.

Aggleton P and Chalmers H (2000) *Nursing Models and Nursing Practice.* Basingstoke: Macmillan Press.

Ball JW and Bindler RC (2006) *Child Health Nursing. Partnering with Children and Families.* Englewood Cliffs, NJ: Prentice Hall.

Barnes K (ed) (2003) *Paediatrics: A guide for nurse practitioners.* Edinburgh: Butterworth-Heinemann.

Bee H and Boyd D (2004) *The Developing Child* (10th edn). Boston: Pearson Education.

Beevers G, Lip G and O'Brien E (2001) *ABC of Hypertension* (4th edn). London: BMJ Books.

Blow WT (2001) *The Biological Basis of Nursing: Clinical observations.* London: Routledge.

Carroll P (1993) Clinical application of pulse oximetry. *Paediatric Nursing* 19(2), 150–151.

Casey A (1988) A partnership model with child and family. *Senior Nurse* 8(4), 8–9.

Casey A (1995) Partnership nursing: Influences on involvement of formal carers. *Journal of Advanced Nursing* 22, 1058–1062.

Childs C, Harrison R and Hodkinson C (1999) Tympanic membrane temperature as a measure of core temperature. *Archives of Disease in Childhood* 80(3), 262–266.

Committee on Blood Pressure Monitoring in Clinical Practice (2004) Medicines and Healthcare Products Regulatory Agency. <http://www.medical-devices.gov.uk> (accessed 14 June 2004).

Crow R, Chase J and Lamond D (1995) The cognitive component of nursing assessment. *Journal of Advanced Nursing* 22, 206–212.

Dhillon R and East C (1994) *An Illustrated Colour Text: Ear, nose and throat and head and neck surgery.* London: Churchill Medical Communication.

Glasper A and Campbell S (eds) (1995) *Whaley and Wong's Children's Nursing*. St Louis: Mosby.

Hanna D (1995) Guidelines for pulse oximetry use in pediatrics. *Journal of Pediatrics* 10(2), 124–126.

Hockenberry MJ, Wilson D and Winklestein ML (2005) *Wong's Essential of Pediatric Nursing* (7th edn). St Louis: Mosby Elsevier.

Jenkins J (2003) Breathing. In: Holland K, Jenkins J, Solomon J and Whittam S (eds) *Applying the Roper, Logan and Tierney Model in Practice*. Edinburgh: Churchill Livingstone.

Lewis H (1999) Chronic cough: Is it asthma? *Archives of Disease of Childhood* 80, 579.

MacGregor J (2000) *Introduction to the Anatomy and Physiology of Children*. London: Routledge.

Mallet J and Dougherty L (eds) (2000) *The Royal Marsden Hospital Manual of Clinical Nursing Procedures* (5th edn). Oxford: Blackwell Science.

Medical Devices Agency (2000) *Blood Pressure Measurement Devices: Mercury and non-mercury. Device Bulletin.* MDA.DB2000 (03) <http://www.mhra.gov.uk/home/idcplg?IdcService=SS_GET_PAGE&ssDocName=COB007350&ssSourceNodeId=235&sstargetNodeId=572> (accessed 21 June 2005).

Nursing and Midwifery Council (NMC) (2002) *Guidelines for Records and Record Keeping*. London: NMC.

Nursing and Midwifery Council (NMC) (2004) *Standards of Proficiency for Pre-registration Nursing Education*. London: NMC.

Orem DE (1995) *Nursing: Concepts of Practice* (5th edn). Mosby, St Louis.

Resuscitation Council (2000) *Basic Life Support Guidelines*. London: UK Resuscitation Council.

Rogers J (1991) Evaluation of tympanic membrane thermometers for use in paediatric patients. *Pediatric Nursing* 17(4), 376–378.

Roper N, Logan W and Tierney A (1996) *The Elements of Nursing Based on a Model of Living* (4th edn). Edinburgh: Churchill Livingstone.

Roper N, Logan W and Tierney A (2000) *The Roper, Logan, Tierney Model of Nursing Based on Activities of Living*. Edinburgh: Churchill Livingstone.

Sims J (1996) Making sense of pulse oximetry and oxygen dissociation curve. *Nursing Times* 92(1), 34–35.

Smith F (1995) *The Nottingham Model*. Oxford: Blackwell Science.

Smith L, Coleman V and Bradshaw M (2001) *Family-centred Care: Concepts, theories and practice*. Basingstoke: Palgrave.

Thorax (2003) British guidelines on the management of asthma. *Thorax* 58 (supplement 1), i1–i92.

Tortora GR and Grabowski SR (2003) *Principles of Anatomy and Physiology* (10th edn). New York: Harper Collins.

Van der Mosel HA (1994) *Principles of Biometric Engineering for Nursing Staff*. Oxford: Blackwell.

Williams C and Asquith J (2000) *Paediatric Intensive Care Nursing*. Edinburgh: Churchill Livingstone.

Wong D, Hockenberry M and Hockenberry-Eaton M (2003) *Whaley and Wong's Nursing Care of Infants and Children*. St Louis: Mosby.

# 8 The Importance of Play

M. DONNELLY AND J. ROBINSON

## INTRODUCTION

Play has been referred to as one of the 'most important aspects of a child's life' (Wong *et al.*, 1999, p. 1171). This chapter will explain the rationale behind this statement, and how the student can contribute to this vital aspect of a child's world. It is intended that by the end of the chapter the student will have gained a greater understanding of the relationship between play and cognitive, social, psychological and emotional development. Chapter 3 of this text also addresses the important issue of play, from a different but complementary perspective.

Bruce (1996, p. 1) describes play as a 'reservoir full of water. The deeper the reservoir, the more water can be stored in it, and used during times of drought.' This time of drought referred to by Bruce could reflect those instances in a child's life when he or she may experience distress due to illness, injury or any other times of physical or emotional trauma. As a result of reading this chapter and working through its scenarios, it is anticipated that you will feel more confident in using play as a form of communication during therapeutic interventions, as a resource that can be used in preparing children for clinical procedures and as a form of distraction therapy.

Developing skills of assessment is an essential prerequisite for those involved in the care of children. Observing how a child plays and interacts can offer valuable information in relation to their condition and relationship experiences (Wong *et al.*, 1999). Developing an understanding of the purpose of play, and what can be expected in relation to engaging in play at various developmental stages, provides the reader with an opportunity to contribute to the multidisciplinary team and assist with appropriate care planning for individual children.

Before examining play in relation to child development and the importance of ensuring that all children are offered the opportunity for play, the immense benefits will be considered. Bruce (1996, p. 3) suggests that play helps children to become 'whole people', who are 'physically healthy, co-ordinated, mentally healthy, manage feelings and ideas and co-ordinate ideas'. If children are permitted to use play during childhood, they can continue to use the resource to

*Caring for Children and Families*. Edited by I. Peate and L. Whiting
© 2006 John Wiley & Sons Ltd

live full lives contributing to the mental and physical well-being of others, becoming creative, sensitive and imaginative adults who have secure relationships with others. Bax *et al.* (1990) remind us that the significance of play to a child's life is not a new phenomenon. Aristotle believed that it was the highest form of human activity; this belief reinforces the need to be able to promote and provide play wherever children are cared for.

The exploration of the importance of play will begin with an understanding of its relationship with physical and cognitive development and what can be expected of children when engaging in play. Cognitive development is discussed in the next section of this chapter.

## COGNITIVE DEVELOPMENT AND PLAY

Those involved in the care of children and their families are constantly reminded that play is not a pointless activity that children participate in during unstructured time (Bee, 1997). Bee goes on to suggest that play is a major factor in relation to cognitive development and that developmental psychologist Jean Piaget's (1952) observations of how children play relate directly to his developmental theories referred to as 'operations'. Bee (1997) suggests there is a correlation between the following operational stages suggested by Piaget.

### SENSORIMOTOR STAGE

This stage occurs from birth to approximately 18 months. At this stage, the child recognises objects through sight, sound and touch. Initially, his or her hands create considerable fascination. This is then replaced by toys presented to the baby, which inevitably are transferred to the mouth for further examination.

### PREOPERATIONAL STAGE

The preoperational stage occurs between 18 months and 6 years approximately. At this stage, the child develops pleasure in the company of other children, although it is not until the latter part of the stage that the child develops the ability to play with other children. Up until approximately 3 years of age, the tendency is to play alongside another child rather than engage in cooperative play.

### CONCRETE OPERATIONAL STAGE

This stage occurs between 6 and 12 years and is when logical thought processes are engaged in. Play becomes more complex with age with children demonstrating an ability to use strategies to problem-solve.

## FORMAL OPERATIONAL STAGE

This final stage is said to occur from 12 years upwards. This is when complex systematic thought processes are used to hypothesise on potential outcomes to problems. Adolescents can be capable of advanced thinking and problem-solving (Bee and Boyd, 2004).

During sensorimotor play, it is suggested that the child of 12 months engages in play through 'exploring and manipulating' objects (Bee, 1997 p. 185). This age group will often place these objects in the mouth, or alternatively shake them or move them along the ground interacting with the environment. Consider the safety implications when selecting suitable resources for a child of this age to play with. Prevention of transfer of infection at this age is a concern, particularly where toys are being played with on a floor of a shared environment (for example a school, play school or clinic) and shared with other children. Ensuring cleanliness of these toys is essential, and the use of communal soft toys, which cannot be easily washed, should be discouraged. Young children can be expected to transfer objects to the mouth, and therefore small items which can cause choking should be made inaccessible, as should broken toys with sharp edges. All those caring for children can play an important role in being vigilant in relation to play resources.

Constructive play tends to occur between the ages of 2 and 6 years. This coincides with the pre-operational stage. It is at this age that children will develop the ability to build using blocks, construct puzzles and make models out of a selection of materials offered to them (Rubin *et al.*, 1983 cited in Bee, 1997). Any selection of appropriate resources in order to continue this type of play either in the clinical or domestic environment will depend on the child's condition and the availability of a play area and the budget for the provision of necessary materials. The child's likes and dislikes are issues that need to be considered when providing for the child's play needs or when advising parents on resources they can provide at home in order to share in the play experience. As this age group falls into Piaget's pre-operational stage, it is worth noting that Piaget (1952) describes this developmental stage as 'centration'. This means that a child of this age has an inability to focus on more than one thing at a time. This point is an important one to be noted by those involved in the planning of therapeutic play for children.

## FORMS OF PLAY

It has been suggested that first pretend play occurs between 15 and 21 months when a child can be observed pretending to feed dolls or drive a toy car. It could be argued that pretend play reflects the theory by Bandura (1989, cited in Bee, 1997) that children learn through observational modelling, and their play may be a replication of what they have observed their parents or a sibling do for them. Consider what information could be gathered by watching a child engaged in pretend play – and particularly in the emotions they may display during this play. This can be observed in a designated play area in the hospital or in a classroom.

The concept of substitute pretend play is displayed between the ages of 2 and 3 years where a child will use an alternative object during play if the necessary object is unavailable. Perhaps he or she may substitute a top from a feeding bottle in the absence of a cup (Bee, 1997). Field *et al.* (1982, cited in Bee, 1997) suggest that this type of play can become quite complex between the ages of 4 and 5 years, when blocks or boxes may be used to construct a car or a house. This highlights challenges for those responsible – such as play therapists and departmental managers – for the provision of resources in a designated play area.

During the preschool period, it appears that children begin to role-play (Bee, 1997). These roles could be 'mums and dads', 'doctors and nurses', 'teachers' or perhaps characters from story books or children's TV characters. Sociodramatic play lends itself to the provision of dressing up clothes, which can be an affordable resource for supervised play areas and in the home (Lindon and Lindon, 1993). Again, this type of play reflects Bandura's (1989, cited in Bee, 1997) 'learning through modelling' theory. Sociodramatic play could be a means by which children re-create previous experiences in their lives. Those experiences may include contact with healthcare professionals. Indeed, the use of uniform and equipment that a child may encounter can be used in this play medium as a means of therapeutic preparation for clinical procedures such as surgery (Douglas, 1993). This type of play could be seen as learning through experience.

Piaget (1952) suggests that the concrete operational stage occurs between the ages of 5 and 7 years. Children at this age may have sustained injuries associated with school activities, perhaps associated with playground activities, and contracted infections following contact with larger numbers of children entering primary school, for example. During this period, it is suggested that children develop the concept of rules or strategies which can be demonstrated intellectually perhaps through simple mathematics, but is also transferable into the arena of play.

It is at this developmental stage, when children play imaginary games and board games (such as Snakes and Ladders) that they learn social rules of authority and how to establish themselves within a social group. These can be offered to children as a means of distraction during stressful times. Although there is evidence of an ability to use strategy at this age, Piaget (1977) argues that children use 'inductive logic', meaning they use their own concrete experiences to formulate general principles, but that they are not adept at 'deductive logic', which requires prediction of an outcome. It could be argued that advances in technology might have influenced these early theories. New technologies, for example complexities of games consoles and computer-generated programs, often involve demonstrating an ability of deductive logic. Many children in the 5- to 7-year age group derive great pleasure from working through the strategies of these games in order to win points. Take some time if you have the opportunity to observe the child on bed rest, who may be using these forms of distraction, and consider the relationship to the concrete operational stage.

Piaget's (1952) final stage of cognitive development is referred to as 'Formal Operational' and refers to the over-12s age group. It is suggested that children and young people at this stage can consider options and possibilities in relation to problem-solving in a systematic way and can engage in deductive reasoning and reach solutions to situations they may not have encountered before. Consider, therefore, the group recreational activities used in relation to outward-bound team-building exercises and sports (knowledge of these areas of play, e.g. favourite teams, can be a useful conversational tool when engaging with young people and can return a sense of control over a potentially frightening experience). Certain computer games have been age-related and involve areas of interests, such as design and simulation, or driving and aircraft-piloting skills. These programs can be used in clinical settings that have access to computer software, such as in designated ward education areas where young people can experience privacy and quiet in an age-appropriate environment.

By considering the cognitive developmental stage of the child requiring provision for play, the student can begin to understand the importance of the appropriate selection of resources which are required if play is to provide stimulation, familiarity, comfort, socialisation and demonstrate respect for the individual child's and young person's needs.


## PHYSIOLOGICAL DEVELOPMENT AND PLAY

Continuing the theme of providing appropriate play resources and environments, a comprehensive understanding of the child's physiological development will again influence planning in this area of care. In relation to the neonate, for example, it is likely that they would be able to focus on a point approximately 20 to 30 centimetres away from them and that they can follow a moving object at the same distance within weeks of being born (Bee, 1997). At the same age, this infant can hear sound 'within the pitch and loudness' of the human voice (Bee, 1997, p. 80). These perceptual skills could be viewed as the child's first developmental understandings of the world around them and the significant people within that world. Having knowledge of these physiological abilities helps the student to consider what could be introduced into the infant's environment to enhance their cognitive development and stimulation. It has been suggested that these introductions must not be beyond their current knowledge of the world or this would be impossible for them to understand (Siegler and Alibi, 2005). Music in an infant's room and cot mobiles appear to be appropriate stimulation for this age group and seem to fulfil the selection criteria for deciding upon the correct attention-getting and attention-holding stimuli so crucial if the stimulus is to be meaningful (Cohen, 1972).

It has been suggested that developmental psychologists use the term 'motor development' when discussing the child's ability to move and use their body in a skilful manner. This can be demonstrated by observing the child at play (Bee, 1997).

By the age of 1 month, it is expected that an infant will be able to lift their head and grasp an object placed in their hand (Bee, 1997). However, the student and healthcare worker must also be aware that objects placed in an infant's hands become rapidly transferred to the mouth as they continue to experience the world around them. Careful attention must be given to the safety implications of selecting suitable toys in order to prevent choking and other accidental injury. If engaging in play with a child of this age, it is essential to remember that as they can only focus approximately 20 to 30 centimetres away from their face objects should be kept within this range, also sudden loud noises may startle them (Reynolds, 1993).

During the period between 6 and 12 months, the infant should be able to sit independently and will reach for objects placed near by. As mobility increases to include crawling and perhaps shuffling on their bottom, this will also enhance their ability to reach objects out of their reach. These newly discovered motor skills can often be carried out at considerable speed; therefore, objects being reached for as an attempt at play must be safe and appropriate (Lindon and Lindon, 1993). This age group experiences immense pleasure from toys that make noises, such as rattles, or activity centres which activate sounds by pressing buttons. They also enjoy being sung to, and musical toys are popular (Reynolds, 1993).

It must be remembered that, while developing an awareness of the normal developmental stages of childhood, consideration must be given to the child who is affected by disability and whose physiological development may not follow the established pattern. This is also true of premature infants and allowances for their play needs should be considered (Lindon and Lindon, 1993).

From 9 months of age, the exploring child becomes ever more mobile – pulling themselves up by furniture, determined to reach interesting objects or toys not intended for them but used by older children (Bee, 1997). This age group enjoys building towers with objects such as play bricks and gains even more pleasure in knocking them down (Lindon and Lindon, 1993). Between 6 and 12 months, children should be permitted the experience of using different textures, shapes and sounds in their play (Reynolds, 1993).

From 12 months of age, the young child will develop the ability to walk and eventually run, increasing their repertoire in relation to play particularly when in the company of other toddlers (Lindon and Lindon, 1993). From the age of

18 months, children have usually learnt the ability to coordinate several motor skills. They enjoy, for example, 'push along' toys (especially those that can be loaded and unloaded with objects such as toy bricks). Toy bikes and cars that can be propelled along by their feet are also popular (Lindon and Lindon, 1993).

Encouraging outdoor play with those aged over 18 months can help to develop physical coordination skills, such as those needed for climbing or riding tricycles. Careful supervision is also required in these arenas because infants do not have the knowledge to determine what objects are safe to climb on (Reynolds, 1993). This age group often enjoys messy play and can engage in simple drawing with large crayons and painting. From the age of 18 months, children enjoy story books being read to them and exploring picture books, all of which add to the variety of play (Lindon and Lindon, 1993).

Motor skills develop further between 3 and 5 years of age. At this age, the child can usually pedal and steer a bike with trainer wheels, catch larger balls and explore small climbing frames and slides, demonstrating increasing muscle development and coordination skills (Reynolds, 1993). An ability to manipulate scissors for cutting (useful during creative play) and the ability to hold a pencil between thumb and first two fingers begins, thus demonstrating an ability to gain more control when drawing or writing (Bee, 1997).

Between 7 and 8 years of age, children become increasingly physically coordinated and develop the ability to ride a two-wheel bicycle and engage in ball games with a degree of skill (Bee, 1997). This transition in scope of play arguably enhances social development as activities of this type often involve teams or groups of other children. Play in relation to team or group activity continues into adolescence in the form of sports, dance and drama; the development of relationships through this type of activity can arguably be essential in relation to the development of self-esteem and self-confidence (Conger, 1991).

## PLAY AND THE CHILD WITH COMPLEX NEEDS AND DISABILITY

When considering and planning for the provision of play, it has already been mentioned that an awareness of the needs of children with disability is essential (Lindon and Lindon, 1993). These authors go on to remind those responsible for facilitating play that limitations in this important aspect of the child's life must be kept to a minimum and that this inevitably means the provision and consideration of appropriate resources for play. These disabilities may encompass a wide range of disorders, including sensory deprivation and physiological and emotional disorders (Lindon and Lindon, 1993). There is a role for provision of play with such children, recognising this activity as 'the universal language of children' (Wong et al., 1999, p. 213).

If children are to truly benefit from the activities of play, the activities chosen must be appropriate to their level of development and ability (Lindon and Lindon, 1993). The philosophy of family-centred care is crucial when planning any care for children, and the concept of working in partnership can itself be a valuable resource when providing specialist resources (Smith *et al.*, 2002). If the child is able to communicate her or his preferences in relation to play these must be taken into consideration in the care planning process (Smith *et al.*, 2002). A consideration of a safe environment allowing for children with visual-field difficulties and mobility difficulties is essential if they are to enjoy the aspects of socialisation and inclusion in the community through play. Consideration must therefore be given to access to the play area in the clinical environment.

Sensory-pleasure play has been found to be beneficial for children with complex needs, such as cerebral palsy, and involves the use of music, light, colour and touch of different materials. These resources can be brought to the child or an environment can be created to include them (Bee, 1997). Tape recorders and a selection of musical tapes, which can be varied by those providing for the child with complex needs, are useful resources along with activity centres, which can be attached to beds and wheelchairs. Mirrored and brightly coloured mobiles should be considered on ceilings of rooms and treatment areas.

## THERAPEUTIC PLAY AND THE SICK AND INJURED CHILD

It has been suggested that there are two main types of play. Normative play, which the child usually engages in spontaneously either on their own or with other children, and therapeutic play. Therapeutic play, however, tends to be purposeful and structured by adults with an intention to maintain the holistic well-being of the child (Huband and Trigg, 2003). This section will focus on the role of therapeutic play.

Whatever environment a child experiences for care, that environment should reflect a consideration to the importance of play in the child's world, particularly as play is said to assist with how a child interprets and understands the world around them (Webster, 2000) and particularly when that world is unfamiliar, such as in the case of the clinical environment. It has been suggested (McClowry, 1988; McClowry and McLeod, 1990) that there are five major influences involved in a child's experience of hospital. They are:

1. developmental stages
2. family separation
3. hospital environment
4. severity of the child's condition
5. existing family circumstances.

Other influencing factors when considering the facilitation of play in a clinical environment can be associated with the cultural attitudes of the family particularly in relation to play and the child's previous experiences (Webster, 2000). Some clinical areas decorate their walls with paintings by children depicting cultural festivals and celebrations from their community engaging in this form of artwork. This can provide familiarity for the child in a strange environment.

The purpose of providing for play in hospital should be to reduce the anxiety induced by a strange environment and to reduce any fear associated with conditions and subsequent clinical procedures (Müller *et al.*, 1995). Therapeutic play can be used as a means of communication between the child and their care providers. It can reduce stress and permit children to express emotions through an acceptable medium (Bee, 1997). By viewing play as a language and not merely an activity, the health carer is equipped with valuable communication tools. Webster (2000) suggests that this tool can be used to develop coping strategies between children and adults responsible for care. By paying careful attention to the child at play, carers can be alerted to their fears, particularly when the child engages in imaginary play with a favourite toy such as a doll or teddy bear.

Often, the child who is playing is coping positively; the child who is not playing and whose presenting condition is such that they would theoretically be able to may be considered to be contemplating their environment and the unfamiliar people in it (Bolig, 1997, cited in Bee, 1997). This could be described as being withdrawn, and strategies to engage the child in personally favoured distractions and activities should be considered.

Within the hospital and community environments the student and healthcare worker may have the benefit of learning specific therapeutic play skills alongside play specialists. Working collaboratively with these other team members is not only related to the development of new and valuable skills but also enables the carer to empower the child to cope with what Bruce (1996) referred to as those times of drought.

The functions of play for the unwell or injured child have according to Bolig (1984) in Müller *et al.* (1995) been said to:

- provide a diversion from what is occurring around them
- allow the child to 'play out problems' and anxieties
- restore normal aspects of life
- aid understanding of hospital events.

When planning the provision of play in order that the above functions can be fully effective, an individualist approach recognising that each child will have different abilities to cope under stress is essential. In relation to the clinical environment, this will be dependent on the child's developmental stage and previous experience (Douglas, 1993). This awareness and ability to recognise potential stressors can assist with predicting and facilitating the play requirements for children in order that they maintain a sense of control over what is happening to them. Douglas (1993, p. 170) suggests that there are certain cues that can assist with these predictions.

*Active or information-seeking versus avoidance*    The child who asks questions and wants to touch the equipment around them in comparison to the child who hides their face and refuses to interact with staff.

*Internal versus external coping methods*    Children who need guided imagery such as relaxation and those who cry out needing distraction and play with preparatory methods.

*Emotionally focused versus problem-focused coping methods*    Children who learn control over and express their feelings and those who engage in problem-solving.

Taking into consideration the above behaviours, it is possible to consider the cognitive developmental stage of the child in relation to these actions. Consider also Bandura's modelling theory (1989, cited in Bee, 1997) and perhaps parental behaviour in relation to health and clinical intervention. It could be suggested that the very young child in particular may take their cues from parental behaviour, emphasising the importance of family-centred care and involvement of the parent in the play experience.

Particular challenges will be encountered with the child displaying poor coping strategies. If this child falls into Piaget's (1952) pre-operational stage, the focus may be centred on a specific aspect of previous care. Being sensitive to the child's individual needs should encourage them to express specific fears, which can then be addressed.

---

**Activity**
*Katie is 4 years old and has been admitted to the children's ward for manipulation under anaesthetic of a fracture to her left arm. In relation to provision of diversion and restoration of normality to her world, what would your considerations be and how would you plan for play provision? Remember to consider her developmental stage and a family-centred approach.*

---

Using play to prepare a child for a clinical intervention has been found to alleviate some of the most stressful aspects of nursing care, but the preparation, as always, must be age-appropriate. Take into consideration previous experiences and be guided by what the child wants to know (Douglas, 1993). Preparatory play can be the arena where children are involved with decision-making, for example would they like to bring their favourite toy to theatre with them? This aspect of play should help with relieving fear and anxiety. In some areas, the preparation can take place in designated pre-admission clinics and home visits, for example as health-promotion activities in schools or on the wards. In the case of emergency admissions, preparation should be considered and provided for whenever appropriate and possible (Webster, 2000).

## PREPARING FOR PLAY

Webster (2000) divides preparation play into three categories:

* medical play
* projective play
* role-play.

It is suggested that medical play uses a combination of real and toy equipment, allowing the child to ask questions and become familiar with what they are likely to experience (Webster, 2000), for example, with the child's permission, a doll or teddy can be used to demonstrate treatment. The child can handle a syringe, dressings, surgical masks, anaesthetic masks and bandages. They can also be invited to become familiar with the sights and sounds of monitoring equipment. A further useful resource for demonstrating nursing procedures has been the use of hand puppets. Children who find it difficult to express frightening feelings such as those experienced with pain have been known to express themselves to the puppet rather than to the person providing the health care (Savins, 2002). Similarly, informative toys can be used with the appropriate age group to demonstrate which part of their body may be requiring treatment (Müller et al., 1995).

Projective play can involve small world play with 'play people' figures. For the child who is overwhelmed by their circumstances and the environment and hides their face from the staff, this form of play can be useful in helping them to work through their fears (Webster, 2000).

Webster (2000) also states that role-play can be an important medium for identifying any confusing or disturbing aspects of child care. The child can dress up to portray adult roles which have become significant to them, for example play clinical uniforms such as a nurse's uniform including surgical masks and stethoscopes can help the child regain control over events. It has been suggested that timing of play preparation is crucial (Webster, 2000). In relation to effectiveness concerning younger children, they appear to benefit from preparation as close to the event as possible, whereas older children can be informed further in advance (Douglas, 1993). It is important to consider at all times the relationship between play and cognitive development. It cannot be emphasised enough that when planning pre-operational play the activities must be age-appropriate if they are to be effective. Piaget's (1952) theory of 'centration' with the pre-operational child should be taken into account and resources must be provided in such a way that the child will understand, if fear and anxiety are to be reduced (Morcombe, 1998).

Using play as distraction is not the same as long-term diversion from unfamiliar circumstances. Instead, distraction should be used in conjunction with preparation to assist with relieving stress before and during treatment, such as suturing and intravenous cannulation (Webster, 2000). Resources can include the child's favourite toy, blowing of bubbles and musical toys (Webster, 2000). The purpose of distraction is for the child to focus on stimuli other than pain, for example attempting to make the experience more bearable. At this time, using the play specialist's expertise may be beneficial (Morcombe, 1998). Methods of choosing distraction should be done in partnership with the family, recognising the parent as a valuable resource in this area of play (Carter, 1994).

Designated areas within clinical environments which are equipped and maintained in accordance with health and safety regulations can provide a haven where children can maintain normalisation and express their anxieties in a cheerful and child-orientated space (Müller et al., 1995). Invasive therapeutic intervention should not take place within the playroom environment if the theme of haven is to be maintained. All areas where treatment is to be performed with children should have attention given to decoration in order to enhance the strategies of distraction; ceiling and wall decorations can be used inexpensively to relieve the fear of unfamiliar environments (RCN, 1998). A designated play area in clinical environments with appropriately educated and experienced staff, such as a play specialist, can promote the value and importance of play to children. Age-appropriate toys, dressing up and messy areas for painting and creativity, gluing and sticking are some examples. Some clinical facilities also provide for outdoor play and a quiet area for storytelling. Working with the play specialist can provide many opportunities for you to develop your skills and understanding of how play can be facilitated, planned for and implemented in a variety of settings where children are experiencing ongoing or future therapeutic intervention (Webster, 2000). Children can use painting and drawing in the play environment as a means of expressing themselves when they find verbal communication difficult or distressing. The multidimensional facets of pain can often be seen in children's painting, and those responsible for the provision of care should observe how children communicate through this medium (Savins, 2002). The value of play and the use of drawings have been discussed in much detail in Chapter 3, which approaches the important activity of play from a different, but interrelated, perspective.

Many of the resources used in the designated playroom are entirely transferable to the bedside and community environment. With forethought and adequate environmental preparation, parents can be supported and advised about resources and how to participate in play with children who may be receiving care at home (Bee, 1997). Adolescents should have their own recreational facilities and be cared for in age-appropriate environments (Taylor and Müller, 1995); the loss of control that can be perceived by the adolescent as a result of admission to hospital (Müller et al., 1995) should always be given due consideration. It could be suggested that possible reactions to hospitalisation by an adolescent might include regression to a more childlike state. Offering distraction through play may relieve some anxiety in this instance (Müller *et al.*, 1995). Creative art play at the bedside can often be welcomed by the adolescent patient, or access to the use of computer games can also be a pleasant diversion.

---

**Activity**

*James is 14 years old and is being cared for in the adolescent ward of the paediatric unit. He has undergone surgery and is recovering two days after orthopaedic surgery on his right leg following a road traffic accident. You have noticed he is quiet and non-communicative. What considerations would you give to helping him through this traumatic experience in relation to diversion?*

---

Visintainer and Wolfer (1975) state that the five areas which cause most anxiety for children and young people being admitted to hospital are:

1. physical harm
2. separation
3. fear of the unknown
4. uncertainty
5. loss of control.

These causes for anxiety are used as guidelines by the RCN (1998) for the care of children in accident and emergency departments and are reflected in the *National Service Framework for Children and Young People and Maternity Services* (DH, 2004).

By offering opportunities for play, you will be providing a valuable aspect of care provision to the patient. Your interventions may relieve anxieties experienced by children and young people who encounter stress in relation to their health. The belief that play should be an integral part of care provision for children is not a new one. This has been highlighted in key policies and guidelines, such as *Welfare of Children and Young People in Hospital* (DH, 1991), the *United Nations Convention on the Rights of the Child* (UNICEF, 1989) and *Children and Young People's Nursing: A philosophy of care* (RCN, 2003). More recently and with a service provision target for delivery of 10 years is the *National Service Framework for Children, Young People and Maternity Services* (DH and DfES, 2004).

## CONCLUSION

The aim of this chapter was to provide the reader with further insight into the essential role of play in a child's life. There are many strategies you could employ (under supervision) that may help to ensure that children can continue to develop, learn and have a more positive experience of health and healthcare provision.

Clinical environments in the hospital and community setting may, for some children, be frightening and threatening. The aim of any healthcare worker is to help alleviate anxieties and fears that the child and their family may be experiencing. Using all available resources, human and material, may go some way to achieving these aims.

Play is an essential aspect of children's and young people's lives. Appropriate and adequate play must be provided for in association with the suggestions made in this chapter as well as those cited in Chapter 3 of this text.

## REFERENCES

Bax M, Hart H and Jenkins SM (1990) *Child Development and Child Health.* London: Blackwell Science.

Bee H (1997) *The Developing Child* (3rd edn.). New York: Longman.

Bee H and Boyd D (2004) *The Developing Child* (10th edn). London: Pearson.

Bruce T (1996) *Helping Young Children to Play.* London: Hodder & Stoughton.

Carter B (1994) *Child and Infant Pain: Principles of nursing care and management.* London: Chapman & Hall.

Cohen LB (1972) Attention-getting and attention-holding processes of infant visual preference. *Child Development* 43(3), 869–879.

Conger JJ (1991) *Adolescence and Youth: Psychological development in a changing world* (4th edn). New York: Harper Collins.

Department of Health (DH) (1991) *Welfare of Children and Young People in Hospital.* London: DH.

Department of Health & Department for Education and Skills (DH/DfES) (2004) *National Service Framework for Children and Young People and Maternity Services.* London: DH/DfES.

Douglas J (1993) *Psychology and Nursing Children.* London: Macmillan.

Huband S and Trigg E (2003) *Practices in Children's Nursing.* Edinburgh: Churchill Livingstone.

Lindon J and Lindon L (1993) *Caring for the Under-8s.* London: Macmillan.

McClowry SG (1988) A review of the literature pertaining to the psychosocial responses of school-aged children to hospitalization. *Journal of Pediatric Nursing* 3(5), 296–311.

McClowry SG and McLeod SM (1990) The psycho-social responses of school age children to hospitalization *Children's Health Care* 19(3), 155–161.

Morcombe J (1998) Reducing anxiety in children in A&E. *Emergency Nurse* 6(2), 10–13.

Müller DJ, Harris PJ, Wattley L and Taylor JD (1995) *Nursing Children: Psychology, research and practice* (2nd edn). London: Chapman & Hall.

National High Blood Pressure Education Programme Working Group on High Blood Pressure in Children and Adolescence (2004) The fourth report on the diagnosis, evaluation and treatment of high blood pressure in children and adolescents. *Pediatrics* 114(2), 555–576.

Piaget J (1952) *The Origins of Intelligence in Children.* New York: International University Press.

Piaget J (1977) *The Development of Thought.* New York: Viking Press.

Reynolds V (1993) *A Practical Guide to Child Development. Volume 1: The child.* Cheltenham: Stanley Thornes.

Royal College of Nursing (RCN) (1998) *Nursing Children in the Accident and Emergency Department* (2nd edn). London: RCN.

Royal College of Nursing (RCN) (2003) *Children and Young People's Nursing: A philosophy of care. Guidance for Nursing Staff.* London: RCN.

Savins C (2002) Therapeutic work with children in pain. *Paediatric Nursing* 14(5), 14–16.

Siegler RS and Alibi MW (2005) *Children's Thinking* (4th edn). Englewood Cliffs, NJ: Prentice Hall.

Smith L, Coleman V and Bradshaw M (2002) *Family-centred Care, Concept Theory and Practice.* London: Palgrave.

Taylor J and Müller D (1995) *Nursing Adolescents: Research and psychological perspectives.* London: Blackwell Science.

UNICEF (1989) *The United Nations Convention on the Rights of the Child.* London: UNICEF.

Visintainer M and Wolfer J (1975) Psychological preparation for surgical patients. *Pediatrics* 55(2), 187–202.

Webster A (2000) The facilitating role of the play specialist. *Paediatric Nursing* 12(7), 24–27.

Wong DL, Hockenberry-Eaton M, Wilson D, Winkelstein ML, Ahmann E and DiVito-Thomas PA (1999) *Whaley & Wong's Nursing Care of Infants and Children* (6th edn). St Louis: Mosby.

# 9 Maintaining Safety

## C. CAIRNS AND L. GORMLEY-FLEMING

## INTRODUCTION

This chapter describes how you can help to provide safe, effective care for children, young people and their carers in three major areas of practice:

- administration of medicines
- infection control.
- moving and handling children

It is important to understand why safety is so important. People expect to be safe when receiving health care, yet providing health care inevitably incurs some element of risk, and 'things will sometimes go wrong' (National Patient Safety Agency (NPSA), 2001 p. 7). Maintaining safety is everyone's responsibility and not just that of managers (HMSO, 1974). Therefore, everyone needs to do everything possible to anticipate, assess and reduce risk. It is everyone's responsibility to report adverse events in order to investigate the causes and learn from them in order to prevent recurrence. Every NHS organisation will have a reporting system, and you should find out what system is in place in your clinical area and how to report an adverse event or near miss.

The National Patient Safety Agency (NPSA) defines an 'adverse event' as 'any event or circumstance arising during NHS care that could have or did lead to unintended or unexpected harm, loss or damage' (NPSA, 2001, p. 13) and 'harm' as 'injury (physical or psychological), disease, suffering, disability or death' (NPSA, 2001, p. 13). Understanding these definitions helps the reader to know what to report. The NPSA also talks about 'near misses', but this is harder to define, since nothing actually happened. An example of this might be an inappropriate prescription which is noticed and changed before the medication is administered.

The NPSA introduced the National Reporting and Learning System in 2003 whereby all incidents and near misses can be reported into a national database, which will be analysed to identify patterns and trends. From these data the NPSA will work with NHS staff to develop practical solutions in order to prevent any recurrence of errors across the NHS.

*Caring for Children and Families.* Edited by I. Peate and L. Whiting
© 2006 John Wiley & Sons Ltd

**Activity**

*If you have been in a clinical area, consider some adverse events you have witnessed or been involved in, and what you have learnt from them.*

*Have you shared this with colleagues?*

*Consider some near misses you have witnessed. What were the significant factors in preventing an adverse event?*

Safe practice is important for students on pre-registration programmes since the NMC requires students to apply knowledge based on the best available evidence, and demonstrate an appropriate repertoire of skills indicative of safe nursing practice (NMC, 2004a).

## ADMINISTRATION OF MEDICINES

### INTRODUCTION

The nursing practice of medicine administration is one that causes increased levels of anxiety for practitioners, and this is considered to be healthy since complacency can lead to errors (Huband and Trigg, 2000). Medication errors do occur and can be serious. Each year a significant number of adverse drug errors occur to infants and children which could be avoided by good practice. A fifth of all clinical-negligence litigation in the UK arises from errors in the use of prescribed medication (Audit Commission, 2002).

Prescribing and administering medicines to children presents a number of challenges to healthcare teams. These include:

- assessing and diagnosing the clinical problem;
- deciding which form of medicine to use;
- determining dosages;
- choosing methods and sites;
- taking into account the child's developmental stage;
- gaining the child's cooperation.

Most errors occur at the prescription phase followed by the administration phase. As the nurse is the one who is most often involved in the administration of medication, he or she is the last barrier between safe practice and serious harm. The administration of medicines is the most common therapeutic intervention that children will receive and is sufficiently important to have its own section in the *National Service Framework (NSF) for Children, Young People and Maternity* (DH and DfES, 2004).

Medicines are an integral part of each of the NSF standards, with standard 10 specifically addressing this issue and identifying the markers of good practice as summarised in Table 9.1 below.

**Table 9.1** Standard 10 of the *NSF (Source: DH/DfES, 2004)*

---

- The best evidence available based on clinical knowledge, safety and cost-effectiveness should be applied at all times to achieve the best health outcomes and to reduce harm in the use of medicine with children and young people.
- Children and young people should have access to equitable, safe, clinically proven and cost-effective medicines in age-appropriate formulas.
- Information is available to all those involved in medication administration, dispensing and prescribing.
- Information for parents, children and carers is timely, up to date and consistent.
- Active partnership is required in all settings with children, young people and parents so that they can be involved in decisions about medicine affecting them.
- All NHS Trusts and Primary Care Trusts must have the use of medicines incorporated into their clinical governance and audit arrangements.
- The contribution of the pharmacist is to be maximised to ensure safety.

---

Students may be involved in the supervised administering of medicines to children if the task is delegated by a registered nurse (RN). However, the student *must* be supervised at all times by the RN. There are two main areas that students need to consider in relation to management of medicines for children.

1. Working with children and families to help them understand about the medicine. This requires an understanding of the specific medicines and their side effects as well as knowledge of the child's development: dealing with refusal and non-adherence.
2. Safe storage and administration of medicine in accordance with legislation, NMC guidance and local policy. This includes the importance of documentation and of monitoring the child for any adverse reaction, evaluation of effectiveness of treatment and adjusting the plan of care accordingly.

These points will be now be considered in turn.

## WORKING WITH CHILDREN AND FAMILIES

Access to safe and effective medicines is essential for children and young people. Parents often take responsibility for this and use over-the-counter medicines for dealing with many episodes of ill health for their children. When a child presents for health care, part of the initial assessment must include finding out whether any over-the-counter or general sales list medicines have been taken. This is necessary so that treatment is not duplicated and to avoid interaction with other prescribed medicines.

Equally, the nurse has an educational role to play in this as parents are often unaware of the side effects of medication purchased over the counter. The assumption is made that, because it was purchased without prescription, the medicine is not very dangerous, which is false, as many children are admitted to hospital following accidental ingestion of medicines that have been purchased over the counter. A study by Chien *et al.* (2003) identified that parents had little awareness of the possible risk of medication purchased over the counter. This highlights the need for education at the time of purchase, the use of patient-information leaflets in a range of languages and continued education in clinical and domestic settings.

Storage of medication in the home must be addressed as an educational need if the incidences of accidental poisoning are to be reduced. Child-resistant containers have helped reduce the mortality rate, but the need for vigilance by parents and carers remains.

## CHILD DEVELOPMENT

The child's development must be considered in all aspects of medication administration. The child is in a constant state of change both physically and psychologically. Their ability to metabolise and excrete drugs varies throughout their childhood (Kanneh, 2002). The child's ability to understand why they are having their medicine can be demonstrated at a young age.

## WHEN A CHILD REFUSES MEDICATION

- Try to establish the reasons for refusal. Use parents/carers and play specialists to try to gauge the child's fears and apprehensions.
- Try to alleviate the problems, provide information, explain timing of medication, use play therapy, discuss alternative ways to administer medicine, and provide rewards such as star charts and certificates. Act as an advocate for the child/family to the medical staff if they are unhappy with medication therapy.
- If the child continues to refuse, discuss with parents whether they wish to continue with medication therapy or how they suggest the medication is administered. In conjunction with the medical team, identify if alternatives are available. Discuss the issue of safety with parents and children. To seek clarity of your role with regard to restraint, access your local policy and the Royal College of Nursing's (RCN, 2002) guidelines on restraint.
- Where parents agree to restraint, the ward manager or designated deputy must be informed. Restraint must be gentle and used for the shortest time possible ('restrain' is a term that the RCN uses to mean 'to limit or control' a child).
- If parents refuse, but the child is legally and ethically competent, or if the parents and child refuse and the absence of the medicine may cause the child actual harm, and is therefore not in their best interests, the multidisciplinary team will need to be consulted.
- Non-adherence is a particular issue and is encountered to varying degrees with the young person. The reason, extent and context of non-adherence must be identified before it can be addressed.

ROLE OF THE FAMILY

The family and carers should be actively encouraged in all aspects of medication administration when their child becomes hospitalised since they may have managed complex medication regimens at home, and may be required to continue treatment initiated during an admission to hospital. Parents and carers often have their own routines and methods for administering medication to their child at home. These should be respected when the child enters the healthcare environment and the nurse should work in partnership with the child and parents to promote this continued practice.

Agreement must be clearly documented in the child's care plan regarding who is going to undertake the administration of medication so as to avoid confusion and errors occurring. Accountability must also be clearly defined. Local policy should reflect family/carer/child's own participation in the administration of medication, with consideration given to the safe storage of the child's own medication. If parents/carers are to undertake new medication administration practice such as intravenous, subcutaneous or nasogastric drug administration, in preparation for going home, then a comprehensive formalised teaching programme, supported by written information and a 24-hour named person to contact must be instigated by the named nurse. Parents/carers should not be pressured into undertaking such procedures. If they do agree to learn the technique, an assessment of the support available should be made to ensure that the child will be safe if the parent who has been taught the skill becomes unable to continue. The nurse should encourage the family to ask questions about their child's medication, and some simple steps can be taken by the nurse to enable this to ensure safe administration in the home upon discharge. This involves the family knowing:

- what the medication is
- what it looks like
- how to administer it
- what device is required to administer it and how to care for them
- how to use it
- what to do if the child misses a dose or refuses to take their medication
- how long the child needs to take the medicine for
- where to seek help and advice
- where to get additional supplies
- how to safely store the medicine.

SAFE STORAGE AND ADMINISTRATION OF MEDICINES

Every organisation will have, as part of their medicines management strategy, a policy for the administration of medicines. This will have been written in the light of current legal and professional requirements. Each policy may have slight variations. For example, some trusts permit single checking of medicines for children, while others prohibit this.

The NMC (2004c) guidelines for the administration of medicines are a set of established principles for safe practice in medication administration and its management. They relate to all registered nurses and should be considered alongside the NMC's code of professional conduct (NMC, 2004b).

These are important to students because although the guidelines state that medication administration must be overseen by an RN (who retains accountability for the administration of drugs) he or she can delegate the responsibility to a patient, parent, student nurse or care assistant. However, the person to whom the task is delegated must be competent to carry out this task and this competence must be reviewed periodically and documented. Before any involvement in any aspect of medication administration, you need to familiarise yourself with the local policy and the NMC guidelines.

The storage of medication is an area of concern for the nurse, whether it is on the ward or in the child's home. Safety is paramount and medication should never be left on lockers or anywhere that the child can reach without the parent or nurse knowing. The drug trolley, drug cupboards and drug fridge must be locked at all times when not in use as. Temperature maintenance (2–5 °C) in the drug fridge should be checked with a suitable thermometer and documented as per Trust policy. Ideally, drug preparation and storage rooms should also have door locks that cannot be opened by children. The keys to the drug trolley should be held by the RN and the trolley should be locked in between each patient administration when performing a drug round if there is any risk of it being unattended at any time.

The regulations for the safe custody of controlled drugs are described in the Misuse of Drugs Act 1971, and Regulations 1973. Drugs must be kept within a locked cabinet and the keys should be in possession of the authorised person, which normally is the ward manager. Records of controlled drugs must be maintained within the controlled drugs register with each drug having its own page within the register. On administration of a controlled drug, records of the patient who received the drug, date, time and amount of the drug and number of ampoules or tablets remaining must be recorded by the person administrating the drug and witnessed by another suitable person, that is the RN or a doctor.

On discharge home, the medication for discharge should be provided in childproof containers, and parents, as part of discharge planning, need to be educated regarding the safe storage of that medication. Childproof containers can be opened by the child; so additional advice is needed, and it is part of the discharging nurse's role to provide this. If medication is to be stored in a domestic fridge, it should be stored in a ridged airtight container, away from food, with the temperature maintained at 2–5 °C.

---

**Activity**
*Find out what the medicines administration policy for your placement area allows and what safeguards are in place to promote safety.*

The administration of medicine is not just a mechanical task and involves a number of members of the multidisciplinary team working together to ensure safe practice, from the correct diagnosis and prescription to the supply of the correct medicine, its safe storage and administration, good documentation, safe disposal, effective monitoring of the child for improvement or side effects and reporting of adverse events, near misses and adverse drug reactions.

In order to gain the necessary competence to be safely involved in this process, you will need to:

- know what specific medicines are used in relation to child health, their therapeutic effect, side effects, precautions and contraindications – lack of drug knowledge has been found to account for 15% of medication administration errors among nurses (Hughes and Edgerton, 2005);
- know how to give medicine by a variety of routes and why each might be chosen;
- know normal dosage range of commonly used medicines and where to obtain this information if required;
- confirm the identity of the child the medicine is prescribed for before administration;
- know why the child is having that specific medicine;
- check that the prescription chart is clearly written, dated, timed and with the relevant information on drug allergies known, child's weight and height and child's name, hospital number, date of birth and address clearly documented;
- check the medicine to be administered and expiry dates;
- ensure medication has been stored correctly and is not visibly damaged or deteriorating (this is particularly important in community settings such as home or school, which may not have the same controls in place as a hospital ward or department and may pose additional safety risks to young children in particular; part of the assessment and preparation for giving medicines to be taken at home should include teaching about safe storage and ensuring that safety in the home is addressed);
- consider the suitability of that medication for that particular child with regard to dose, route, timing and preparation and their overall plan of care;
- accurately calculate the amount of medication to be administered and recognise whether your calculation is correct;
- provide emergency action and contact medical staff promptly in the event of an adverse drug reaction (some medicines require special care when given off hospital premises and some may only be suitable for administration on such premises due to their high-risk nature);
- accurately and clearly document the administration of the medicine immediately, even if this procedure has been delegated to the child or their parents (best practice advocates that you observe the child swallow the medication before documenting; when supervising or delegating to a student, the RN must clearly countersign the signature of the student);

- provide the family and child with adequate information about the drug, its therapeutic value, side effects and any other relevant information (this is a shared responsibility with the prescriber);
- monitor the child for benefits, reporting any side effects that become apparent, and advise the carers of what to look for and what action to take should they occur.

## POINTS TO CONSIDER IN THE SAFE ADMINISTRATION OF MEDICINES

1. Wash hands (see 'HAND HYGIENE', p. 183) before and after handling medicines.
2. The medication administration procedure should not be interrupted at any stage. If interruption is unavoidable, the administration of the medication's process should recommence from the beginning.
3. The nurse allocated to the care of the child for that particular period of duty should be the one accountable for all medication administration for that child. In the case of a student or healthcare assistant being that person, he or she must know which RN on duty is supervising their practice, so that they may be approached to administer medication to the child.
4. Never prepare drugs in advance and leave them sitting on lockers – this is waiting for an accident to happen. If it is oral medication, you must make sure that you have witnessed the child swallow their medication before you sign that it has been given. If it is rectal, you should make sure that the child has retained the suppository for at least 20 minutes (Galbraith *et al.*, 1999).
5. Be competent in drug calculations and know where to seek help if you need more practice.
6. Never camouflage medication in food or drinks – what will you do if the child refuses to finish the food or drink? How can you document that they have received the correct dose in this situation? You need to refer to the UKCC's (2001) guidance on disguising medication for further reading on this area.
7. Use correct equipment – oral syringes should be used for oral medication of small volumes, not other syringes (DH and DfES, 2004).
8. Gain the child's cooperation: ensure they understand and never threaten them. Praise and reward will lead to a much more pleasant experience for all concerned.
9. Protect the child's clothing with a tissue or bib and position the child in such a way as to prevent aspiration and choking (Watt, 2003).
10. Dispose of all waste as per Trust policies, taking special care if the waste has to be transported to another site (e.g. from home to base for disposal) and ensure you have safe travel containers.

**Table 9.2** The six *r*'s of safe administration of medication

| |
| --- |
| The *right* medication |
| The *right* patient |
| The *right* time |
| The *right* route |
| The *right* dose |
| The *right* to refuse |

## SAFE ADMINISTRATION

It is imperative that the nurse observes the six rules (the six *r*'s of medication administration shown in (Table 9.2) in order to ensure safe practice. From the time the child reaches an age of basic understanding, informed consent becomes a very real issue, hence why the right to refuse has been added to this list. Understanding how medication errors and near misses occur provides the practitioner with important information on preventing future medication errors. Refusal has been discussed earlier in this chapter.

## THE LEGAL FRAMEWORK

There are a number of aspects of legislation affecting the administration of medicines to children. These are grouped around the supply and administration of the medicines themselves (Medicines Act 1968, Misuse of Drugs Act 1971, Medicinal Product: Prescription by Nurse etc. Act 1992 and the Children Act 1989/2004).

The key points from the legislation mentioned above are summarised here. The pharmacist working with your team will be able to provide more information.

### Medicines Act 1968

This comprehensive piece of legislation provides the legal framework for the manufacture, licensing, prescription, supply and administration of medicines. It classifies medicine into the following categories:

#### *Prescription-only medicines (POMs)*

- These are medicines that may only be supplied or administered to a patient on the instruction of an appropriate practitioner (a doctor, dentist or from an approved list for non-medical prescribers). Oral antibiotics and antiepileptic medication are examples of POMs.

*Pharmacy-only medicines*

- These can be purchased from a registered Primary Care pharmacy provided that the sale is supervised by the pharmacist, for example some antimalarial medications and antifungals.

*General sales list medicines*

- These can be purchased from retail outlets as they do not need to be prescribed or require the supervision of a pharmacist, for example paracetamol and ibuprofen.

(Over-the-counter medicines is not a legal classification but a generic term that covers both general sales list and pharmacy-only medicines.)

## Misuse of Drugs Act 1971

This legislation is concerned with controlled drugs and categorises them into five separate schedules. RNs are particularly concerned with schedule two and as such should familiarise themselves with this act.

## Medicinal Product: Prescription by Nurse (etc.) Act 1992

This Act allows certain groups of nurses, midwives and health visitors to prescribe a limited range of medication and products from a limited formulary or as a supplementary prescriber. This is a growing area of practice, and you may be working alongside nurses who are either independent or supplementary prescribers.

---

**Activity**
*How might nurse prescribing assist the care a nurse may provide to a child?*

---

## Children Acts 1989/2004

Two aspects of these Acts are very important to consider in relation to the administration of medicines.

1. The need to establish who holds parental responsibility (and so who can give legal consent/make decisions).
2. The Acts reinforce the child's involvement in decision-making and partnership with parents.

## UNLICENSED MEDICINES AND THEIR USE IN CHILD HEALTH

The DH and DfES (2004) have addressed the issue of the use of unlicensed medication in children with an outline plan to resolve this issue by 2014. There are many reasons why some medicines are not licensed for use in children.

1. Clinical trials have not been performed on children.
2. Medicines might be used for rare illness.
3. There are too few children in need of medication to warrant a clinical trial.

Medicines that are unlicensed or 'off-label' are often necessary in child health as there may be no substitute available. In this situation, the child and parents should be informed. As a nurse, you need to be satisfied that there is acceptable evidence for using the medication as intended and that you have sufficient information to administer the medication safely (NMC, 2004c). The Royal College of Paediatrics and Child Health (2000) has produced generic patient information leaflets explaining why it is necessary to use unlicensed medication for parents and children.

---

**Activity**
*What does the term 'off-label' mean? Who would you ask to talk to a family asking for more information about this?*

---

## DRUG CALCULATIONS

Basic maths skills are fundamental when it comes to administering drugs to patients. Incorrect calculations are a significant source of drug errors. While an element of human error will always exist in healthcare practice, the ability to correctly calculate a drug dose and articulate units of measurement is absolutely essential to the safe administration of medication and one way to reduce medication errors.

Golden rules for calculating drug doses are as follows.

- Look at the prescription and identify what drug you want and how much of it.
- Identify what you have (the amount) on the medication bottle/ampoule/table.
- Convert all weights and volumes in the equation to the same units, e.g. micrograms, milligrams or millilitres.
- Write down each step and change only one unit at a time so as to reduce the risk of error.
- When everything is in the same units that you need, use the formula:

$$\frac{\text{What you want (the dose prescribed)} \times \text{what it is in (the volume available)}}{\text{What you have (the strength of the medicine available)}}$$

For example, a child is prescribed 80 mg of paracetamol. The bottle of paracetamol suspension has 120 mg in 5 ml. How many ml will you give the child?

$$\frac{80\,\text{mg} \times 5\,\text{ml}}{120\,\text{mg}} = 3.33\,\text{ml}$$

- If a second person is checking the medication with you, you should both independently calculate the dose and then compare answers.
- Does it look logical? If not, recalculate.
- Remember, calculators are not foolproof and are no substitute for your mathematical ability. While they are designed to improve accuracy, you must be competent at mental arithmetic.

---

**Activity**
*Calculate the following:*
*A child has been prescribed 200 micrograms of morphine. There is 1 mg in 1 ml. How much will you draw up?*

---

This section has considered the administration of medications for children from a safety perspective with consideration given to the child's development, the role of the family and refusal of medication. Other areas that have been addressed are the legislative frameworks that govern nursing practice and the practicalities of medication administration. While medication errors may never be eliminated from practice, the risk of them occurring in the first instance must be reduced. This is only one aspect of safe practice and the next sections will seek to address some others.

## INFECTION CONTROL

This chapter is not an infection-control text but is designed to give the reader a sound basis for practice based on current knowledge. Infection control is, and always will be, an important feature of every healthcare worker's role, especially those who have significant direct contact with children, young people and their carers. It has been observed that clinical staff, and healthcare assistants in particular, have a significant role to play in educating other professionals such as medical staff (Spencer *et al.*, 2000), and it is the intention here to give an overview of the issues and how good practice can be ensured.

CONTEXT/BACKGROUND

At the time of writing, politicians of all political parties are responding to public concern about the cleanliness of hospitals and the increasing and seemingly unstoppable prevalence of methicillin-resistant *Staphylococcus aureus* (MRSA). While there is no firm evidence to link so-called dirty hospitals with the spread of infection, common sense and our perception tells us that there may be a link and we may, therefore, acquire an infection in a 'dirty' hospital. All healthcare workers have responsibility for aspects of the prevention and control of infection and in keeping premises clean and tidy. Those working with children and young people have a particular role to play in keeping the environment clean and tidy so that cleaning staff can do their job properly. There is, however, good evidence based on case reports and outbreak investigations of a link between 'dirty' environments and hospital-acquired infections. If poor infection-control techniques and practice are adopted by nurses and healthcare assistants working in clinical areas when there is a child with an infection, an outbreak of disease may occur and this may have serious consequences.

The National Audit Office (NAO) (2000) found that around 9% of patients acquire an infection during their hospital stay. This costs the NHS around £1 billion and causes at least 5000 deaths each year. Furthermore, some of these infections could have been prevented if good practice had been in place, thus reducing distress for patients and saving the NHS money which could then be spent in other vital areas. MRSA is a significant infection, and it is estimated that the problem is now so serious that 10% of the general population is carrying MRSA (NAO, 2000). Therefore, nurses and healthcare assistants working in all settings need to understand the principles and practice of good infection prevention and control, whether they work in hospital or community settings. Standard principles for the prevention of healthcare-associated infection in primary and community care have been produced (National Institute for Clinical Excellence (NICE), 2003) to complement the guidance issued to organisations providing care in hospitals.

There are many ways in which staff can help to reduce the incidence of cross infection. These include learning and practising skills such as effective hand hygiene and aseptic technique and by contributing to patient and family education.

## HAND HYGIENE

Hand hygiene is a vital factor in the prevention and control of infection (DH, 2003) and is fundamental in protecting both the client and the healthcare worker from acquiring micro-organisms, which may cause harm. Hands can become contaminated through direct contact with children and young people, indirectly by handling equipment or through contact with the general environment. Because contamination is not usually visible, and we cannot see the transfer of contaminants or organisms, we may become complacent about how clean our hands are.

Micro-organisms found on the skin are classified as transient or resident. Transient microbes are acquired from many environmental sources through hand contact and are very easily passed on to the next surface that is touched. Resident micro-organisms live within the epidermis and serve to protect the skin from more harmful bacteria. Infection is most likely to come from transient microbes.

Hands should be washed whenever there is a chance that they may have become contaminated, and certainly before and after physical contact with

**Table 9.3** When hands should be washed

Hands should be washed:
- immediately you arrive at work
- before and after examining each client
- before putting on gloves for clinical procedures
- after touching any instrument or object used on a client
- after handling blood, urine or other bodily fluids
- after removing any kind of gloves
- after using the toilet
- before preparing/eating food
- after contact with your nose or mouth
- after contact with dirt, dust or grease
- before and after medication administration
- before leaving work.

patients, their food, invasive devices or dressings (Pratt *et al.*, 2001). Table 9.3 lists occasions when you should wash your hands.

Hand washing may seem a simple task and one which is engaged in from childhood, but, to be effective, a thorough and rigorous technique is required.

**Levels of hand hygiene**

Hand washing should involve a vigorous, brief rubbing together of all surfaces of your lathered hands; the hands are then rinsed under a stream of running water. There are three levels of hand hygiene.

*Social hand washing*   This removes transient micro-organisms and is appropriate, for example, before eating. Washing with liquid soap is adequate, although alcohol hand rub may be used for social hand washing if the hands are visibly clean.

*Hygienic hand cleaning*   This removes transient and some resident micro-organisms by using agents with disinfectant properties such as alcohol hand rub. This level should be used after contact with blood and all bodily fluids.

*Surgical hand washing*   This removes all transient and the majority of resident micro-organisms. Agents with disinfectant properties are used in conjunction with a longer hand-washing procedure (Infection Control Nurses Association, 2006). This technique would be used, for example, prior to an invasive procedure such as a lumbar puncture.

The process of drying your hands is an important part of the hand-washing technique as micro-organisms transfer more easily on to wet surfaces than on to dry ones.

Disposable paper towels should be used to dry the hands, as they not only dry the skin effectively but they will also remove any transient micro-organisms and dead skin cells which are loosely attached to the surface of the hands. These paper towels can then be disposed of into a domestic waste bin. One of the challenges of community nursing is to carry out good hand hygiene in a home that may not appear clean. Community nurses should therefore be equipped with an individual supply of appropriate solutions such as alcohol gel and paper towels.

Sore, chapped hands also increase the risk of infection as bacterial counts are raised in damaged skin. Any cuts or broken skin should be covered by a water-proof dressing. While many hand-hygiene products on the market do contain moisturisers, applying moisturising hand cream may further protect hands. Communal tubs of cream must be avoided as the contents may become contaminated.

Although hand hygiene is the most effective method of decontaminating your hands, you may also find a supply of alcohol gel beside each bed space in hospital as part of the Clean*your*hands campaign (National Patient Safety Agency (NPSA), 2005) to which most hospitals have signed up. A risk assessment needs to be done in areas where children are cared for in order to balance the risk of accidental ingestion of gel against the risk of cross infection. You may also be given a personal supply of gel for use in circumstances where it is not possible to wash your hands before touching the patient. All staff working in community teams should have their own supply of gel to carry with them at all times.

UNIFORM

Uniforms are an important vehicle for the transmission of organisms. The issue is currently a matter for debate as a strict uniform policy requires the provision of adequate changing facilities, sufficient uniforms and a reliable laundry service. You should check the uniform policy of your Trust to find out what it says. Some of the important things to find out are the following.

1. What am I allowed/expected to wear? In general, you should wear a freshly laundered uniform (whatever form that takes) each shift. Clothing should be appropriate for the clinical area, allow full movement for safe moving and handling (see below) and permit good hygiene practice. Sleeves should be short or rolled up, and other items of clothing, such as ties, should also be avoided as they are known to harbour microbes and should not be worn for clinical contact. Hair should be worn off the collar and neatly tied away from the face in a manner that does not require frequent adjustment. Pony tails are not acceptable as they can fall forward over the shoulder and could contaminate a wound.
2. Do I have to wash my own uniform (or my own clothes if worn) and, if so, at what temperature? In order to provide effective decontamination, uniforms should be washed at a minimum of 60 °C for 10 minutes or 71 °C for 3 minutes. Domestic washing machines cannot achieve this standard.

3. What jewellery is acceptable? In many Trusts, wedding bands are permitted but no other rings. Stoned or heavily faceted rings, bracelets, facial jewellery, earrings (other than single studs) and wristwatches *must not* be worn by staff undertaking clinical procedures as they are reservoirs of infection since they prevent effective hand cleaning.

4. What if I have religious or cultural reasons for wearing specific items of dress such as long sleeves or head coverings? In this case, discussion will take place with your manager and the infection-control team in order to balance the infection-control risks against your religious or cultural needs. Where these items are permitted, they must be laundered regularly at the required temperature to ensure decontamination.

5. Can I go outside the hospital precinct in my uniform? You should not go into commercial premises in your uniform (however casual it is) and should change as soon as possible after the end of your shift. If you have to travel in your uniform, you should cover it completely – a short jacket is not sufficient. You should also avoid close contact with children or pets at home in your uniform before going to work as they may transfer organisms on to your uniform that you then transfer to the workplace.

6. Healthcare staff who wear their own clothes need to refer to and adhere to their Trust's uniform policy or dress code.

A common-sense approach and knowledge of good practice in the prevention and control of infection will help to minimise the chance of transferring organisms between you, your patients, your family and others. Infection control not only serves to protect the patient but also the healthcare professional.


## TRAINING/LINK NURSES

You should be given training in infection control both by the university or training organisation and in clinical placement areas. If you do not have this training, ask for it. As a minimum, this should include hand hygiene, universal precautions and any special procedures relevant to your clinical placement, such as caring for children who are immuno-compromised for any reason, or those who have infections.

Most teams have an infection-control link nurse. Find out who the link nurse for your team is and what learning resources are available to you. They will be knowledgeable in most aspects of the prevention and control of infection and will have access to the expertise of the infection-control team if required.

You should also take time to find out where the infection-control policy is found in each placement area and familiarise yourself with this. Although the principles of infection prevention and control are universal, each Trust has its own way of translating this into practice. There will also be local policies in clinical areas to supplement the Trust's policy and account for the special needs of children, young people and their families in that area.

Other policies you should also be familiar with are those for hand hygiene, decontamination, needlestick injury, management of sharps and disposal of clinical waste. This is particularly important for staff working outside hospital premises, as they may need to transport waste. You should also check the admission policy for your clinical area and find out under what circumstances new patients are isolated and if swabs are to be taken or not. If children and young people are to be isolated on admission pending clear swab results, you should remember the psychological and social impact this may have on them and their families.

Another policy of particular concern to staff working with children, young people and their families is decontamination. Every piece of equipment used by more than one patient must be cleaned between each use (Pratt *et al.*, 2001). Special care should be taken in the cleaning of toys and games as well as clinical equipment. More and more clinical equipment is provided for single use only to avoid the need for chemical or other types of cleaning, but some items, such as infusion pumps, do need to be cleaned between patients. Items designated for single use only by the manufacturer must never be reused. Check whether an item is for single use or for use by a single patient. If an item can safely be cleaned and decontaminated, you should find out what the local procedure is and how to get an item cleaned or decontaminated. Your clinical area may have an equipment link nurse who will be able to help; otherwise, your mentor, supervisor or team leader will know. Items should always be cleaned in accordance with the manufacturer's instructions, which is generally wiping with a cloth dampened with detergent in solution. Using alcohol wipes on some items of equipment causes damage to the fascia over time and should not be used unless specified by the manufacturer.

Toys and games are vital to a child's well-being and development while in hospital (Chapter 8). Toys should not be shared unless they are cleaned properly, or, if they cannot be properly cleaned, they should be kept for one child only. This also applies to shared highchairs and buggies. Advice can be obtained from the local infection-control team, and there may be written advice in the infection-control manual.

Children and young people are in hospital for the minimum time necessary and therefore the turnover of patients is very fast. You should find out who is responsible for cleaning beds between patients and how this is done. Failing to do this properly increases the possibility of transmitting organisms between patients.

## ASEPTIC TECHNIQUE

Infection can be freely introduced at any time during an invasive procedure or when the integrity of the skin is broken. An important method of preventing infection during this time is through adopting an effective aseptic technique.

Opinion varies as to the best technique, and you should find out which aseptic technique is applied in your clinical area. Whichever technique is used, it should be appropriate for the location (home, school or hospital) and the task. It may also be possible for the family and/or child to be taught the technique if this is appropriate and they wish to learn to do so. If this is the case, there will be a local process for achieving and documenting this.

The underlying principle of asepsis is to reduce infection risk through preventing the transmission of organisms into wounds or other vulnerable sites. This is achieved through only allowing 'sterile' items to come into contact with such sites. Rowley (2001) points out that in most environments it is impossible to maintain a truly sterile environment owing to the presence of atmospheric micro-organisms and therefore argues for the use of a clean procedure such as the 'aseptic non-touch technique' (ANTT).

Whichever technique is used, it is important to know the principles of asepsis and the rationale for the technique chosen in your clinical area. You should not vary the technique without discussing this with senior colleagues as this is confusing for children and their families and can also make the audit of infection rates difficult to monitor.

ANTT (Rowley, 2001) is commonly used in children's clinical areas and may be taught to you in your clinical areas. The main features of ANTT are as follows.

- **A**lways wash hands effectively
- **N**ever contaminate key parts
- **T**ouch non-key parts with confidence
- **T**ake appropriate infective precautions (e.g. eye protection, disposal of waste).

Some clinical areas, based on their considered opinion of the evidence and an assessment of the risk, use a more traditional aseptic procedure. If this is the case, you will be taught the relevant technique.

### What should I do?

Do not undertake aseptic technique until you have been taught to do so and are competent in the procedure. Follow the procedures you are taught and set a good example for others. Do not be afraid to challenge those who do not follow the correct procedure. If you do not feel able to do this, speak to someone more senior.

If you have any suggestions for improving practice in this area, make them to your mentor, supervisor or team leader.

The prevention and control of infection requires knowledge and skills that are used in performing a number of tasks and interactions with children, young people and their families and is therefore also a consideration in safe moving and handling.

# MANUAL HANDLING OF CHILDREN

## INTRODUCTION

Moving and handling is defined as:

> any transporting or supporting of a load (including the lifting, putting down, pushing, pulling, carrying or moving thereof) by hand or bodily force. (Health and Safety Commision, 1992 and Health and Safety Executive (HSE), 1998a, p. 1)

Moving and handling infants, children and young people is an integral part of nursing practice, and competent handling is an essential component of holistic care – but the nurse needs to be acutely aware of the risk of manual handling.

The risk of musculoskeletal damage and injury must be considered by all who work in the clinical environment, irrespective of the activity being undertaken. Twenty-four per cent of NHS staff regularly experience back pain, and one in four nurses will have taken time off work at some time with a back injury sustained at work (DH, 2004).

The need to look after one's back is paramount, and this has been addressed through training, the introduction of medical aids to assist with manual handling, safe-handling policies and campaigns to promote safe working practices. Safe-handling policies often state that nurses should not lift at all (RCN, 2002). This does not fully reflect the needs of the infant and child in hospital.

Height-adjustable cots are not readily available. Parents often accompany their child to hospital and a bed for the parent alongside the child's bed or cot often restricts access for the nurse to perform nursing care, particularly at night-time when he or she is trying not to disturb the parent or child.

When working with infants and children, much time is spent working at the level of the child and holding infants and children. This is either to perform nursing care such as feeding or medication administration or to comfort them. In these circumstances, the 'no lifting' principle advocated by the guidelines needs careful consideration. This type of moving and handling is often referred to as therapeutic handling since it is necessary in order to be able to deliver patient care. It would seem terribly cruel to leave an unaccompanied child crying in a cot when a cuddle would pacify them. Education, having height-adjustable beds and cots and individual 'child specific' risk assessment forms will enable the practitioner to determine appropriate safeguards whether in hospital, community or home environments.

Before undertaking the activity of moving and handling, you need to understand the musculoskeletal system and how this functions. This will be covered in an anatomy and physiology textbook.

Safe-handling practice can be defined as an ergonomic approach to handling people, encouraging independence where possible and the appropriate use of equipment while promoting independence (Brown-Wilson, 2001).

**Table 9.4** Regulations and codes of practice for manual handling

Health and Safety at Work Act 1974
Manual Handling Operations Regulations 1992 (amended 1998)
Management of Health and Safety at Work Act 1992 (amended 1999, see below)
Management of Health and Safety at Work Regulations 1999
Provision and Use of Work Equipment Regulations 1998
Lifting Operations and Lifting Equipment Regulations 1998
Reporting of Injuries, Diseases and Dangerous Occurrences Regulations 1995
RCN's Code of Practice for the Handling of Patients 2002

This section will address safe practice in relation to the principles of moving, handling and positioning, the legislation that governs practice, some of the issues particular to moving and handling with infants and children, the use of equipment and training.

## LAW RELATING TO MOVING AND HANDLING

The duty of care owed to children is decreed by both statute and common law, whether in the hospital or community setting. Legislation in the form of statutes and regulations place a duty on the employer to ensure that employees avoid the need to lift manually if at all possible (HSE, 1998c). The law relating to moving and handling consists of various Acts of Parliament and approved codes of practice (Table 9.4). You must also comply with Trust and local policies and protocols associated with safe moving and handling.

### Health and Safety at Work Act 1974

Employers are obliged under this principal piece of UK legislation to ensure, so far as is reasonably practicable, the health and safety of their employees while at work. The obligations of the act can only provide an effective guarantee of health and safety if the workforce is prepared to cooperate with the employer (Montgomery, 2003). Therefore, the employee's duties are to take reasonable care of their own and other people's health and to cooperate with their employer to enable them to perform their duties, for example use hoists and pat slides and attend annual training in manual handling.

### Manual Handling Operations Regulations 1992 (amended 1998)

Employees' responsibilities for their own safety are clearly set out in these regulations as are those of employers. In summary, employees need to:

- adhere to appropriate safe systems of work as laid down for their safety;
- have access to safe and proper equipment to minimise risk of injury;

- cooperate with their employer on health and safety issues, such as by following local policies, use equipment where provided and report harm;
- ensure that their activities do not put others at risk.

Employers need to:

- avoid the need for manual handling as far as reasonably practicable;
- assess the risk of injury from manual handling that cannot be avoided;
- reduce the risk of injury from manual handling as far as reasonably practicable, e.g. provide appropriate equipment and have policies and protocols in place.

### Management of Health and Safety at Work Regulations 1992 (amended 1999)

These regulations place an obligation on the employer to undertake risk assessment of the workplace regularly and act accordingly.

### Provision and Use of Work Equipment Regulations 1998

These place requirements on the employer (Dimond, 2004) to provide:

- suitable work equipment for the task;
- information, instruction and training on the equipment;
- proper maintenance of equipment and controls and control systems.

### Lifting Operations and Lifting Equipment Regulations 1998

These regulations came into force in December 1998 and apply to all premises and work situations that are subject to the Health and Safety at Work Act 1974.

In summary, the key points are that:

- any lifting must be planned, supervised and carried out by a competent person(s), e.g. picking an infant up from a cot, moving monitoring equipment from a storage area to a child's bedside;
- training of employees in the use of equipment must be given;
- all lifting equipment must be suitable for the purpose, be sufficiently strong and stable;
- before being used for the first time, lifting equipment should be thoroughly examined;
- lifting equipment and accessories such as slings must be marked with appropriate information for their safe use;
- lifting equipment must be examined with service records maintained by a competent person at agreed intervals;
- defective equipment must be reported promptly.

**Reporting of Injuries, Diseases and Dangerous Occurrences Regulations 1995**

Any work-related death, accident, personal injury or sickness where the employee is absent for more than three days must be reported to the HSE under this regulation. Records of all such accidents must be kept for at least three years.

In addition to the UK legislation, unions and professional organisations have reinforced the rights and responsibilities of employees with a more practical perspective. For example, the RCN has produced a code of practice for the handling of patients (RCN, 2002).

This advocates the elimination of hazardous manual handling but recognises the difficulties of this for staff working with infants and children, suggesting that the risk of injury can be reduced by considering the ergonomic issues and the use of full risk assessments. It places responsibilities on the employer to adhere to all of the above legislation but also to implement measures to ensure employees have health checks and that uniforms allow for unrestricted movements when handling patients. The employee has a duty to inform the manager if there:

• is a lack of equipment or staff;
• are any environmental hazards;
• are defects in the equipment;
• are injuries or accidents;
• are any illnesses or disabilities that affect handling capacity.

The Human Rights Act 1998 should also be considered in all moving and handling situations. The child and young person's human rights to have their dignity protected and their physical integrity maintained cannot be stressed enough. Health and safety legislation may not be enough to adequately protect nurses and carers from the human rights claims of the patients or their families (Fullbrook, 2004).

RISK ASSESSMENT

One of the most important things that will help keep children and their carers, both professional and family, safe during unavoidable moving, handling and positioning activities is risk assessment. This is particularly important for the family and other social carers whose needs may be neglected, which often results in poor technique leading to injury and progressive damage.

Child-specific risk-assessment forms should be utilised when assessing the child either in the hospital or community setting. The HSE (1998a) advocates the formal assessment of all procedures involving handling a load using a 'Risk Assessment Framework', as does the RCN (2002). This is called an ergonomic risk assessment and should form part of the child's assessment and care plan, thus being available for reference and used as and when required. When such an assessment is done at a young age, it must be repeated as the child grows or their condition changes. Similarly, it must be reviewed as the physical mobility of the carer changes through age.

Ergonomic risk assessment should assess the following.

- **The Task:** How much can the child do independently? How often is this task required? What postures are involved? Does it need to be done? Does it involve stooping, twisting or holding? How many staff are available? Does it involve transferring the child over a distance? Is there risk of sudden movement?
- **The Individual:** Has the person been trained? Is the person assisting trained? Is there any danger to pregnant women? Is there any danger to those with a health problem/recent injury? Is the individual appropriately dressed – including footwear? Has the weight and height of the individual been considered for this task? Has the individual performed this procedure with this patient before?
- **The Load:** this can be either the object or the patient.
  - **Object:** Is it heavy, bulky or an unusual shape? Is it difficult to grasp? Is it hot, wet, cold or sharp?
  - **Patient:** What is the matter with the child? How ill are they? What is their weight? Can they weight-bear? Are they weak? Are they in pain? Are they frightened or do they have behavioural problems? What is their developmental stage? What is their level of consciousness? Is there any sensory loss? Is there any equipment attached to the child? Can the child communicate? Are there any language, cultural or gender considerations? Will the family be involved?
- **The Environment:** Is there enough space to move freely? Is lighting adequate? Is the floor space cluttered, wet or uneven? Can the clutter be moved? What is the temperature of the room? Is the equipment readily available, used safely and in good repair? This is particularly important in the child's home where conditions may be less than ideal and modifications or special equipment such as hospital-style, adjustable-height beds, hoists or additional storage space may be required before the child can be safely cared for at home.

## PRINCIPLES OF MOVING AND HANDLING CHILDREN

Adherence to the principles of moving and handling are paramount if we are to ensure the safety of the patient, their family members, our colleagues and ourselves. You must adhere to your Trust's policy on manual handling. The key principles of safe moving and handling infants, children and young people are as follows.

1. Do not lift if at all possible.
2. If a child needs to be moved, appropriate equipment should be utilised where necessary. It is important to communicate the procedure to the child and family beforehand. The child and family need to be involved in discussions and their preferences identified.
3. Encourage the child to help as much as they possibly can themselves; ultimately, this may avoid the need for manual handling. It is important that the child feels that they are not being transported from one place to another with little or no say. For example, a child on bed rest might be able to do a bridge when they require a bedpan or having their clothes changed. If transferring a child from a bed to a chair, they may well be able to edge their way to the side of the bed, thus completing the first part of the process, or a sliding sheet may be placed beneath them to help them move more independently. Any independence that can be encouraged is important as it will increase the child's feelings of security, well-being and self-esteem.
4. Do not try to perform other tasks while lifting or handling a child.
5. There is no such thing as a quick lift or a 'simple assist'.
6. Many children are too heavy to be lifted and equipment is required.
7. If lifting cannot be avoided, the risk needs to be assessed. Refer to the child's care plan. Identify handling hazards and regularly review this care plan.
8. Consider the task, individual, load, environment and equipment before progressing with handling the child, ensuring the correct skills are possessed by all those involved in the handling process.

## DEVELOPING GOOD PRACTICE IN MOVING AND HANDLING CHILDREN

There are many incidents in clinical practice where the infant, child and young person will require assistance to either move, alter their position or require handling for therapeutic interventions. Crucial to safe moving and handling practices, a number of issues need to be considered throughout the span of childhood.

### Physiological development

For the infant, with immature neurology resulting in lack of muscle tone (Bee, 1998), the carer will be in complete control of the infant's moving and handling. The infant can quickly identify a favourite position. For the sick infant, handling might need to be kept to a minimum so that their condition will not deteriorate. All carers need to be aware of specific positions and handling required by the infant and this should be documented in their plan of care. Equipment can be requested and provided on an individual-needs basis at short notice.

Lack of muscle tone can remain a problem for the child with special needs; equally, their muscle tone can increase, which presents a challenge in terms of position, moving and handling. When moving a child with a lack of muscle tone, it is important to remember that they are likely to be unstable and difficult to grasp (Huband and Trigg, 2000). These children will be totally dependent on you for moving.

For the child who has a neurological impairment with abnormal movements such as athetoid or ataxic movements, stability is required when they are being moved or handled. These children may have an exaggerated startle reflex, thus certain points on their bodies may need to be controlled (Eckersley, 1993). Handling needs to be steady and firm to avoid painful muscle spasm and harm occurring to the child. Consultation with the child's parents is paramount to ascertain correct moving technique, as is reference to their plan of care. Involvement of the physiotherapist is also essential in planning safe moving for the child with neurological impairment in both hospital and community settings.

Muscle tone and control develops as the child continues to grow, but muscle strength and bulk may still be an issue prior to puberty, hence the inability of children to move themselves as easily as adults.

Coordination ability must also be considered with the young child when trying to promote independent moving. It is helpful to practise techniques with children before any surgical procedure that is going to result in a period of immobility. Encourage the child to help as much as they possibly can. This will improve their technique and increase their confidence with any equipment.

---

**Activity**

*You need to transfer Robert, aged 9 years, from his bed to his chair as he wishes to attend the playroom. Robert has spastic quadriplegia and is totally dependent on his carers for all his needs. He has increased muscle tone and weakness and increased reflexes. Robert dislikes being moved.*

*First of all, you are going to refer to Robert's risk assessment and identify how many people are required to help, the type of equipment required and how Robert reacts. Robert will be hoisted into his chair so you need to ensure that you have been trained in hoisting, are able to apply Robert's slings safely and ensure safe transfer of Robert from his bed into his chair while adhering to local policy. Robert will probably voice his concerns, and you will need to ensure that he remains safe during hoisting. This can be achieved with the help of another staff member. Once Robert is in his chair, you must remember to ensure his safety harness is in place securely and that you tidy away the hoist to maintain a safe environment for the other patients.*

**Activity**

*Jane is 13 months of age and has cerebral palsy with a lot of muscle spasm. She loves being cuddled and this really settles her when she attends her respite day centre. Jane should have a risk assessment performed and her plan of care should have been discussed with her parents on her admission to her day-care facility and documented. Jane may be carried astride her carer's hips as this has been shown to reduce muscle tone, but this is not for the long term as it may put the carrier's spine into a twist position if she is carried like this for too long. Equally, this may not be very good for Jane's hips. Alternatively, she may be carried with her arms hanging down over her carer's back, facing her carer with her legs held slightly apart (RCN, 2002). Jane's specific method of handling must be known to all of the team so as to prevent harm to Jane and to her carers.*

**Psychosocial development**

The use of developmental stages is a means of identifying the achievement of milestones. This must be considered in safe moving and handling. Interventions based on desired behaviours can be planned in partnership with the child and family, according to their developmental stage. Some tasks may be beyond the child's ability at that point in time due to their having not yet reached that particular developmental milestone. Children may or may not be able to visualise what is required of them in relation to their participation in moving and handling but may grasp what is required by a demonstration or by careful explanation.

It must be borne in mind that developmental regression as a result of hospitalisation or illness frequently manifests itself. Equally, children and young people in hospital may be reluctant to cooperate as a result of not understanding what is asked of them: fear, being in a strange environment or that moving may exacerbate pain may be some of the reasons for this. Good communication, outlining the rationale for the actions required along with negotiation and appropriate nursing care should alleviate this, enabling cooperation and adherence to procedures.

## FAMILY INVOLVEMENT

The philosophy of child healthcare practice is based on the concept of family-centred care and partnership. Parents often wish to continue with their child's care while in hospital and the benefits of this are well documented (Casey, 1993; Smith *et al.*, 2001).

In the case of moving and handling, this then becomes a shared responsibility between the professionals, the non-professionals and the parents as a result of negotiation. It has been identified that parents give priority to their child's needs over any risk to their backs when lifting and handling (Griffin and Price, 2000), and therefore any risk assessment must take account of parents' needs.

With the length of stay in hospital being reduced and the emphasis being placed on care in the community, preparation for discharge with regard to moving and handling is paramount for the safety of the child and parent/carer. Interprofessional discussions need to take place prior to discharge to ensure the home environment has been assessed and is suitable, with alterations made before discharging the child. Training of the parents and provision of equipment must also have taken place prior to discharge and, ideally, this should be revisited once the child is home. Regular contact with a named professional, usually a community children's nurse, should be established.

---

**Activity**

*How would you negotiate parental involvement in the moving and handling of their child? What information would you need to know? Is the fact that they have not received moving and handling training an issue?*

---

## TRAINING AND EQUIPMENT

Prior to undertaking any moving and handling tasks or the use of any equipment, it is essential that all staff have been trained and assessed as competent in these areas. The 'Clinical Negligence Scheme' for Trusts (NHS, 1996) has an established set of standards to manage risk and promote good practice. Under this scheme, moving and handling training is mandatory for all staff, including those in training and temporary workers. It is your responsibility, however, to access training and to ensure that you are fit for practice.

Training is also necessary in the undertaking of patient risk assessments and the completion of such documentation. This may be a formal programme or taught in the clinical area by an experienced professional, such as a nurse, physiotherapist or occupational therapist. It must be considered that training is an integral aspect of patient safety and needs to be undertaken at regular intervals (for example annually) and when moving to specialist areas of practice. You need to refer to your Trust's policy to identify training requirements and be able to access the manufacturer's instructions for all equipment being used. The manufacturer's instructions must be read prior to use. There is a huge variety of equipment available and familiarisation with equipment in the clinical or community setting is essential prior to use.

Equipment is provided to ensure the safe practice of manual handling. Some of the most common equipment used is listed below.

- Hoists and slings (electrical and mechanical). These eliminate the need for manual handling. They are used for transferring to chair, bed, bath, from floor or over a distance.
- Stretcher hoist. Used to lift someone who is in a semi-reclined or supine position, e.g. from a bed on to a treatment couch.

- Standing hoist, dual purpose so it can be used as a standard mobile hoist also. Used to transfer person from sitting to standing, e.g. toileting, and to move someone while standing. Promotes some independence.
- Ceiling track hoist. Overhead hoist that is either manual or mains powered and removes the need for manual handling.
- Profiling bed or cot. Consists of three or four platforms that can be brought together into a profile shape. The patient can use the controls to adjust their own position to be able to sit up or lie down independently.
- Sliding sheet. A sheet or netting with hand loops for the carer to grab. Used to transfer patient from a bed to a trolley or changing position from side to side in a bed.
- Monkey pole. Fixed to the top of the bed, within reach of the child enabling them to bridge (raise their buttocks off the bed) for toileting purposes. This is not suitable for younger children as they may not have the coordination and upper body strength to perform this movement. It is often used for children on bed rest or those in traction of the lower limbs.
- Rope ladder. This is attached to the end of the bed and allows children to pull themselves into a sitting position.
- Hand blocks. These are blocks with hand grasps that are placed on either side of the child in the bed, enabling them to pull themselves up the bed. The child must have good upper arm strength and coordination to be able to use these.
- Turning discs. These are made from a slip-resistant material and consist of two discs that rotate in opposite directions. They are used (fabric disc only) to change a patient's position in bed by placing it under their buttocks or when standing (hard disc), placing them in a better position to move independently perhaps.
- Transfer board (Patslide®). A hard board suitable for lateral transfer of a child from a bed to a trolley or vice a versa.
- Bath board. Suitable for children who can take their own body weight through their arms, allowing the child to sit on the board in a bath.

It is appropriate that you are familiar not only with all equipment before you begin to use it but also with maintaining that equipment (safe storage, appropriate servicing and keeping it clean) ready for patient use. If equipment is not available, it needs to be requested. It is the manager's responsibility to provide equipment, ensure staff are trained in its use and that it is maintained in accordance with the manufacturer's requirements and the Trust's policy. In relation to cleaning equipment, reference should be made to the manufacturer's instructions and local policy.

## IDENTIFYING UNSAFE PRACTICE

Unsafe moving and handling practices have no place in the clinical environment. This must not be tolerated as it is placing the patient, the healthcare staff and carers that are involved in the procedure at risk of injury. Clinical risk incident forms need to be completed if you witness poor practice. The ward/clinical manager, clinical facilitator/placement support nurse and link lecturer must also be informed as required and appropriate action taken to ensure that best practice is implemented.

## CONCLUSION

Moving and handling infants, children and young people is a complex procedure with many areas where potential harm could occur both to the child and their carers. Each child is unique and requires an individual plan of care in relation to their moving and handling requirements. Nurses need to satisfy themselves that they have the knowledge and skills to perform this plan before ever contemplating moving or handling a child. Annual updating is essential to keep abreast of new techniques, regulations and equipment.

This chapter has outlined:

- the knowledge and skills required for safe practice in the care of children and young people in relation to the administration of medicines;
- prevention and control of infection;
- moving, handling and positioning.

It has described the legal and professional frameworks which underpin practice in each of these areas.

In order to become competent and confident in these areas, you should work with your mentor to develop the knowledge and skills in a range of settings. You should make sure that you are aware of developments in the legal and professional frameworks and any changes in practice arising from research or other evidence. Do not do anything unless the guidelines for practice are met and you have had prior teaching.

## REFERENCES

Audit Commission (2002) *A Spoonful of Sugar: Medicines management in the NHS.* London: Audit Commission.

Bee H (1998) *Lifespan Development* (2nd edn). London: Addison-Wesley.

Brown-Wilson C (2001) Safer handling practice for nurses: A review of the literature. *British Journal of Nursing* 10(2), 108–114.

Casey A (1993) Development and use of the partnership model of nursing care: In Glasper A and Tucker A (eds) *Advances in Child Health Nursing.* Harrow: Scutari Press, pp. 183–189.

Chien C, Marriott JL, Ashby K and Ozanne-Smith J (2003) Unintentional ingestion of over the counter medications in children less than 5 years old. *Journal of Paeditrics and Child Health* 39, 264–269.

Department for Education and Skills (DfES) (2005) *Children Act 2004*. London: HMSO.

Department of Health (DH) (1989) *Children Act 1989*. London: HMSO.

Department of Health (DH) (2003) *Winning Ways: Working together to reduce health-care associated infection in England. Report from the Chief Medical Officer*. London: DH.

Department of Health (DH) (2004) *Back in Work Campaign*. London: DH.

Department of Health & Department for Education and Skills (2004) *National Service Framework for Children, Young People and Maternity Services. Standard 10*. London: DH/DfES.

Dimond B (2004) *Legal Aspects of Nursing* (4th edn). Harlow: Pearson Longman.

Eckersley PM (1993) *Elements of Paediatric Physiotherapy*. Edinburgh: Churchill Livingstone.

Fullbrook S (2004) The human right to dignity v. physical integrity in manual handling. *British Journal of Nursing* 13(8), 462–468.

Galbraith A, Bullock S, Manias E, Hunt B and Richards A (1999) *Fundamentals of Pharmacology: A text for nurses and health professionals*. London: Addison Wesley/Longman.

Griffin S and Price V (2000) Living with lifting: Mothers' perceptions of lifting and back strain in child care. *Occupational Therapy International* 7(1), 1–20.

Health and Safety Commission (1992) *Management of Health and Safety at Work Regulations: Approved code of practice*. London: HMSO.

Health and Safety Executive (HSE) (1995) *Reporting of Injuries, Diseases and Dangerous Occurrences Regulation*. London: HMSO.

Health and Safety Executive (HSE) (1998a) *Lifting Operations and Lifting Equipment Regulation*. London: HMSO.

Health and Safety Executive (HSE) (1998b) *The Provision and Use of Work Equipment Regulations*. London: HMSO.

Health and Safety Executive (HSE) (1998c) *Manual Handling: Manual handling operations regulations* (2nd edn). London: HMSO.

HMSO (1974) *The Health and Safety at Work Act 1974*. London: HMSO.

Huband S and Trigg E (2000) *Practices in Children's Nursing. Guidelines for hospital and community*. Edinburgh: Churchill Livingstone.

Hughes R and Edgerton EA (2005) First do no harm: Reducing pediatric medication errors. *American Journal of Nursing* 105(5), 79–84.

Infection Control Nurses Association http://www.icna.co.uk (accessed May 2006).

Kanneh A (2002) Paediatric pharmacological principles: An update. Part 3. *Paediatric Nursing* 14(10), 36–43.

Montgomery J (2003) *Health Care Law* (2nd edn). Oxford: Oxford University Press.

National Audit Office (2000) *Improving patient care by reducing the risk of hospital-acquired infection: A progress report*. Report by the Comptroller and Auditor General, HC 876 Session 2003–2004. Norwich: TSO.

National Health Service (NHS) (1996) (Clinical Negligence Scheme) Regulation XI 1996 No 251; amendment regulations SI 2002 No 1073. London: DH.

National Patient Safety Agency (2003) *Seven Steps to Patient Safety: A guide for NHS staff*. NPSA: NHS.

NICE (2003) *Infection Control: Prevention of healthcare-associated infection in primary and community care*, London: NICE.

NPSA (2001) *Doing Less Harm: Improving the safety and quality of care through reporting, analysing and learning from adverse incidents involving NHS patients – Key requirements for health care providers*. London: NPSA/DH, version 1a.

NPSA (2005) Clean*your*hands campaign. <http://www.npsa.nhs.uk/cleanyourhands> (accessed 13 June 2005).

Nursing and Midwifery Council (NMC) (2004a) *Standards for Pre-registration Nursing Programmes*. London: NMC.

Nursing and Midwifery Council (NMC) (2004b) *The NMC Code of Professional Conduct: Standards for conduct, performance and ethics*. London: NMC.

Nursing and Midwifery Council (NMC) (2004c) *Guidelines for the administration of medicines*. London: NMC.

Rowley S (2001) Aseptic non-touch technique. *NT Plus*, 97(7), vi–viii.

Royal College of Nursing (RCN) (2002) *RCN Code of Practice for Patient Handling*. London: RCN.

Royal College of Paediatricians and Child Health (2000) *The Use of Unlicensed Medicines or Licensed Medicines for Unlicensed Application in Paediatric Practice*. London: RCPCH.

Smith V, Coleman M and Bradshaw M (2001) *Family Centred Care: Concepts, theories and practices*. Basingstoke: Palgrave.

Spencer R, Perry C, Connelly E and Bowden E (2000) Students learn infection control on the job. *British Medical Journal* 321, 573.

United Kingdom Central Council (2001) Disguising Medication. *Register* Autumn, 37.

Watt S (2003) Safe administration of medicines to children: Part 2. *Paediatric Nursing* 15(5), 40–44.

# 10 Accident Prevention

## M. DONNELLY AND B. KELL

## INTRODUCTION

The purpose of this chapter is to provide an understanding of the incidence of childhood accidents and how they can be prevented. Childhood developmental stages and behaviours which influence the occurrence of accidents will be discussed, along with what affecting factors need to be taken into consideration when participating in the prevention of accidents through health-promotion activities. In order to illustrate the challenges encountered by healthcare services, statistical evidence will be provided for consideration and reflection; particularly in relation to the essential part they could play in reducing incidence of accidents by safeguarding and supporting children through the work of accident prevention.

The *Oxford English Dictionary* (2005) defines an 'accident' as an 'unintentional or unfortunate harmful event'. Indeed, the *National Service Framework for Children, Young People and Maternity Services (NSF)* adopts this interpretation and addresses the need to act upon the prevention of accidents to children under the heading of 'unintentional injury' (Department of Health and Department for Education and Skills (DH and DfES), 2004). The influence of the *NSF* and other significant government initiatives in relation to accident prevention will be discussed later in the chapter.

It must be remembered that, when caring for children, young people and their families, there are expectations that the care provided will be of a professional standard, ethical and legal. The law expects the interest of the child to be of paramount importance in the provision of care (DH, 1989), and therefore it could be argued that the prevention of childhood accidents could be viewed as a legal obligation.

Try to aim to develop an awareness that childhood injury necessitates a high profile in relation to healthcare provision for the following reasons: injury is the main cause of death in childhood in the UK; it can result in serious ill health and disability; and the incidence and results of injury impact on cost for the NHS, society, families and children (Towner, 2002).

*Caring for Children and Families*. Edited by I. Peate and L. Whiting
© 2006 John Wiley & Sons Ltd

In order to consider the impact of accidents on children, young people and their families an overview of statistical evidence is now provided; consider this evidence in relation to your current work activities.

## SOME ACCIDENT RATES

- Between 1998 and 2000, 1003 children died in England as a result of accidental injury (DH, 2002a).
- In 2000 there were 320 283 road accident casualties in the UK; 16 184 were child pedestrians (0–15 years) (DH, 2002b).
- In 2002 in the UK 26 000 children under 5 years of age were taken to hospital with suspected poisoning, and an estimated 1 000 000 children aged 5–14 attended hospital following an accident outside the home (this did not include road traffic accidents) (DH and DfES, 2004):
  - ○ ingestion of iron supplements causes great concern and is associated with an increased mortality rate in children under the age of 5. Iron supplements can be found in households where pregnant women live and are used in the prophylactic treatment of iron deficiency anaemia (McCrea and Bates, 1999);
  - ○ other toxic substances ingested by children include paracetamol, ibuprofen (often in elixir preparation), bleaches, disinfectants and detergents (Bates, 2001).
- Substances of low toxicity ingested by the under 5s which result in attendance to hospital services such as accident and emergency departments include the following:
  - ○ pencil 'leads', these are made from graphite not lead;
  - ○ wax crayons from the UK originating from reputable companies and produced for children would not be hazardous;
  - ○ emulsion paints, PVA (polyvinyl) glue and wallpaper paste (Bara, 2002);
  - ○ under 5s are also known to ingest soil, compost and plants and plant food, animal food products usually intended for cats, dogs and fish, and cosmetics (this is by no means an exhaustive list but reflects a young child's keenness to explore their environment, particularly once they become mobile) (Bara, 2002).
- Between 1992 and 1999 there were 90 fatal drownings involving children under 5 years of age. These related to the following water features: garden ponds, swimming and paddling pools and other water containers (Department of Trade and Industry (DTI)).
- Every year over 100 000 people require hospital treatment as a result of accidental burns or scalds, and 45% of all severe scalds and burns are suffered by children under the age of 5 years. Of these accidents, 50% take place in the kitchen (DTI, 1999). These injuries result not only in serious physical harm but also in long-term psychological damage (DTI, 1999).

# INJURIES AND DEVELOPMENTAL STAGES
# OF CHILDHOOD

In order to prevent accidents and provide effective health-promotion advice, an understanding of the physiological, psychological and cognitive development stages of childhood and adolescence is needed. A sound knowledge of the developmental stages of childhood and adolescence may help the health professional to anticipate certain types of accidental injury, and provide the healthcare worker with an ability to anticipate potential harm and be proactive in accident prevention.

From the outset, children are vulnerable to accidents owing to their immature developmental stage and natural curiosity of the world around them; although the newborn infant may not have extensive motor skills at birth, they normally have impressive perceptual skills (Bee and Boyd, 2000).

At birth, the baby is expected to be able to focus on a point approximately 10 to 15 centimetres from them. This allows them to recognise their mother's and father's faces in comparison to other faces. Within a few weeks, the baby will be able to follow an object with their eyes (Bee and Boyd, 2000). The newborn can recognise human voices and will quickly identify their main caregiver in this way. They also have an ability to recognise four basic tastes:

- sweet
- salty
- sour
- bitter

and will recognise familiar smells such as that of their mother or father (Bee and Boyd, 2000).

The infant is totally dependent on the care giver for the maintenance of their safety. Indeed, the United Nations refers to the Declaration of the Rights of the Child (1924) within the Convention on the Rights of the Child (1990) stating that 'the child, by reason of his physical and mental immaturity, needs special safeguards and care' (UNICEF, 2002).

An example of accident prevention directed at parents can be found in the work carried out by the Foundation for Sudden Infant Death (FSID). The FSID, in its 'Baby zone' website (<http://www.sids.org.uk/fsid/babyzone1.htm>), promotes the avoidance of parents sleeping with babies, as there is significant risk of the sleeping adult accidentally suffocating the infant. By discussing the work of professionals such as health visitors and midwives, you will become aware of how this type of accident prevention is being addressed in the community through individual education and also established parenting classes.

By 2 months of age, the infant is developing significant motor skills which include trying to grasp nearby objects with the hand (Bee and Boyd, 2000). Consider, therefore, the potential for accidents, such as scalds, when a baby is being held by an adult who is also holding a hot drink. The reason may be to reach the cup. Incidents such as this can have serious consequences in the form of scalds, as the adult will be unable to extricate the child's grip with both hands occupied, and by attempting to pull the cup away boiling fluid may be spilt. The child is at a physical development stage where 'letting go' has not yet become an acquired skill; cognitively the child will not be aware of the potential danger.

Motor skills can be divided into loco/gross motor skill and manipulative/fine motor skills. Between 1 and 3 months, the infant will begin to lift their head and sit with support. This is known as gross motor skills (Bee and Boyd, 2000). The ability to hold an object placed in the hand at this age, or reach for an object by grasping with the whole hand, is referred to as fine motor skills (Bee and Boyd, 2000). Between 4 and 6 months, the infant is becoming increasingly mobile and will demonstrate gross motor skills of rolling or shuffling, sitting independently and then progress to crawling, resulting in an ability to reach for and grasp objects not necessarily intended for them (Bee and Boyd, 2000). Consider, therefore, the increased risk of ingesting inappropriate or toxic substances or rolling off a bed if left unattended. Also consider raising the parent's awareness of the child's environment and its attendant potential hazards.

In addition, at this stage there appears to be evidence of the child trying to understand their environment by exploration. Piaget (1977), an eminent developmental psychologist, suggests that a child's cognitive development can be divided into schemes known as 'operations'. They are as follows:

- **Sensorimotor stage** (from birth to 18 months): responds to the world through what their senses present; there appears to be no plan attached to how they respond to presented stimuli.
- **Preoperational stage** (from 18 months to approximately 6 years): understands that objects exist even though they cannot be seen and therefore will attempt to search for objects, which can lead to accidents such as climbing on to chairs or work surfaces to reach shelves or cupboards.
- **Concrete operational stage** (from 6 years to approximately 12 years): develops an ability to devise strategies to overcome problems and understand the world around them.
- **Formal operational stage** (from 12 years onwards): at this stage, the child develops deductive logic and has the ability to consider consequences of actions even though they have not been experienced yet; this becomes crucial if the adolescent is to make safe choices in relation to risk-taking activities.

The developing motor skills of the child extend to standing and walking between the age of 12 and 18 months (Illingworth, 1991). The potential for a greater range of accidents inevitably occurs. The added height of being able to stand allows the child to reach objects that were once unattainable. Potential problems include the flexes of kettles hanging over kitchen work surfaces and handles of saucepans on stoves that can now be reached and tipped with boiling contents on to the exploring child. These hazards will now require constant supervision and should be moved out of the child's reach.

As the child's confidence in their ability to mobilise continues, their natural curiosity in relation to their environment will lead them towards staircases in the house and areas in gardens such as pools. The potential for injury in these areas is obvious. It may be appropriate to raise parental awareness regarding the high risk of serious injury and consequently empower parents to prevent accidents occurring through delivering appropriate health-promotion education in the home or clinical environments where families access services such as child and family clinics, GP surgeries or accident and emergency departments. The use of stair gates, the filling-in or gating of ponds and pools are examples of the sort of advice that would need to be discussed.

By the time the child reaches 2 years of age, they can be expected to develop further independence. This physical independence manifests itself in an ability to climb stairs confidently, turn door handles and unscrew lids off containers (Illingworth, 1991). Clearly, the ability to anticipate the child's capacity for travelling independently on foot and investigating, once inaccessible, areas and containers increases the potential for accidents, particularly in the form of ingesting toxic substances. Although containers of toxic substances such as household cleaners and medication usually have childproof lids, in the case of the determined and curious child these might not always be effective. It has been noted that the child becomes skilled at an early age with the use of available 'tools' in the solving of problems (Siegler, 2005); therefore, advice in relation to the locking-away out of reach of any potential harmful substances is clearly the safer option. A constant awareness and sensitivity is required regarding the parents' capacity and ability to ensure safety within the home environment. As with any care provision, a robust assessment of need would be required in order to safeguard the health and welfare of the child (DH, 2000). This is discussed further later on in this chapter.

From approximately the age of 7 years, the child's motor skills extend to include the ability to ride a two-wheel bicycle or to use a skateboard. It is also at this stage that their independence may be extended to playing outside but still close to the home environment. However, although their perception of dangers could be expected to be considerably further developed in comparison to the much younger child, the environment beyond the home will offer new dangers that they will not have previously experienced.

If the older child is to cope safely beyond the confines of home, the child must learn further rules about the extended environment if they are to avoid accidents on the roads, injuries caused by falling from bikes and swimming injuries. Specific accident-prevention initiatives will be discussed later in this chapter. You may find yourself involved in accident-prevention activities with the older child within the school. The collaborative practice between health and education is essential if injury and mortality rates are to be reduced in childhood, and is also part of the vision within standard one of the *NSF* (DH and DfES, 2004).

The developmental stages of adolescence are sometimes referred to as the 'Tasks of Adolescence' (Taylor and Müller, 1995, p.44) and include the following:

- adjusting to a rapidly changing physique and sexual development;
- achieving a sense of independence from parents;
- acquiring the social skills of a young adult;
- developing necessary academic and vocational skills;
- achieving a sense of oneself as a worthwhile person;
- developing an internalised set of guiding norms and values.

Young people at this developmental stage provide further challenges in the field of accident prevention. Road traffic accidents are a significant cause of death among young people and have been highlighted as an area for attention by the Government (DH and DfES, 2004).

Accidents in this age group can include sports injuries caused by involvement in contact sports such as football or rugby or more high-risk extracurricular club activities such as skiing, canoeing, sailing, climbing and mountain walking – all which are valuable in developing independence and social and academic/vocational skills. However, the nature of adolescence and its association with risk-taking activities results in admissions to accident and emergency departments with injuries linked to the effects of experimentation with drugs and alcohol (Holt, 1993) and injuries associated with fighting and road traffic accidents (either as pedestrians or drivers).

It has also been suggested that a proportion of adolescents who take part in what could be deemed irresponsible behaviour resulting in accidents have an apparent inability to perceive long-term consequences, some of which may be fatal either to themselves or others (Hendry and Kloep, 1996), for example the adolescent car driver who drives at speed or under the influence of alcohol or drugs.

Facilitating the personal safety of the young person presents new challenges, and becoming involved with youth group workers in clubs, schools, colleges and established community drop-in facilities known to be accessed by young people can enhance understanding and participation in health-related activities.

---

**Activity**

*Imagine you are accompanying a health visitor on a first-time visit to a mother who has just had her second baby, who is now 2 weeks old. As well as Mum and the newborn infant, you meet 1-year-old Amy, who has recently become mobile around the furniture. Taking into consideration the developmental stages of these children, what environmental observations would you be making in order to assess safety in relation to accident prevention?*

*What operational stage of development is Amy at, according to Piaget? What are Amy's motor skills likely to include? Have you considered kitchen work surfaces, hot fluid, stairs, household cleaners and family medication?*

---

# FACTORS AFFECTING INCIDENCE OF ACCIDENTS

This section will consider in a little more detail the factors which affect the incidence of accidents in childhood. The reason for exploring these is that in doing so it is possible to identify relationships between them; this knowledge can then guide the giving of appropriate information and support to children and their families to prevent accidents in the future. It is important to acknowledge from the start that these factors cannot be seen in isolation but impact upon each other.

---

**Activity**
*Consider the following situation:*
*Jack is 18 months old and has reached all his developmental milestones. He lives with his mother in a sixth-floor local authority flat. Jack's mother is 18, has recently lost her job and is worried about how she will cope without the income from this. She is now receiving benefits.*

*What factors do you think could place Jack at risk of accidents occurring?*

---

Within this scenario and in relation to Jack you may have identified the following factors.

- Jack is male.
- Jack is 18 months old.
- Jack is at a developmental stage where he can probably walk well and run carefully, push and pull objects and pick up small items immediately on sight with a delicate pincer grip. Jack can walk upstairs with a helping hand and possibly even downstairs. He is also now able to explore his environment energetically with increasing understanding but has no sense of danger.
- Jack's home environment could pose some risks to him.
- Jack lives in a single-parent household, facing the social and economic difficulties of his mother's low socio-economic group.

## GENDER

In terms of gender, being male appears to be a significant factor in childhood accidents as boys are approximately twice as likely as girls to have accidents (Child Accident Prevention Trust (CAPT), 2005). In 2003, Haynes *et al.* in their study looking at injuries in 5- to 14-year-old children identified boys as having a 35% greater likelihood of accidents and also found that the risk of injury appeared to increase with age with each year adding 7% to the risk. But why is gender a contributing factor? Towner *et al.* (2005) suggest a range of reasons (Table 10.1).

**Table 10.1** Reasons why gender may be a contributory factor to accidents
*(Source: Towner* et al.*, 2005)*

- different rates of physical development
- motor coordination
- spatial ability
- cognition and intellectual development
- gender differences in behaviour (e.g. risk-taking, peer pressure)
- different forms of play and levels of independence
- different levels of supervision and freedom of activities
- exposure to different environments

DEVELOPMENTAL STAGE

As can be seen from Table 10.1, Jack's age and developmental stage will affect his chances of an accident occurring. A useful tool for this is Sheridan's (1997) illustrated charts of children's developmental progress, which identify different developmental stages segregating posture and large movements, vision and fine movements, hearing and speech and, lastly, social behaviour and play.

Jack at 18 months is more likely to have an accident in the home environment, whereas school-aged children are more likely to be involved in road traffic accidents. This is supported by Home Accident Surveillance System (<http://www.hassandlass.org.uk>) data, which collates data in terms of the accident mechanism by age and sex. Age and developmental stage are closely linked; so, although Jack may be well supervised by his mother, as infants and young children tend to have greater levels of supervision and control over their activities, as he grows and develops the seriousness of injuries may increase due to his increased levels of participation in activities that could result in accidents. One reason given for this is that development is advancing so rapidly in the child that he or she is often able to encounter risks without actually being able to understand that they are dangerous or even how to avoid them (Pless, 1993). The link between a child's developmental stage and accidents can best be seen by exploring the types of accidents that occur in specific age ranges. CAPT has produced an excellent resource specifically raising awareness of the various types of risks children may encounter at each developmental stage.

**Activity**
*If Jack was not 18 months old but 14 years old, what would then be the risks posed?*
    *Remember to think about this in relation to his gender and developmental stage.*

In the activity you may have identified some of the following aspects:

- more likely to incur a road traffic accident, owing to increasing independence;
- exposure to different environments;
- may be involved in greater risk-taking behaviour such as substance misuse/abuse;
- influenced by peer pressure.

## SOCIO-ECONOMIC FACTORS

Socio-economic factors are difficult to define as they are made up of many components, such as social class, family income, maternal education, family structure and accommodation to name a few (Towner *et al.*, 2005); some of these will be explored in more depth later in this chapter. Towner *et al.* (2005) identify a number of socio-economic factors in terms of risk of injury (Table 10.2).

Socio-economic factors are a key feature of childhood accidents at all ages and in all developed countries including the UK (Kendrick and Marsh, 2001; Haynes *et al.*, 2003). It is important to note that the risk of injury is strongly related to socio-economic disadvantage as was identified by Laing and Logan (1999) when exploring patterns of unintentional injury in childhood and their relationship to socio-economic factors. Socio-economic disadvantage can be ascertained using tools that measure deprivation. The Jarman index, for example, uses a formula to express the health needs of communities being served by health authorities (Jarman, 1983), while the Townsend index uses proxy measures of deprivation, such as not owning a car or electricity disconnection (Townsend *et al.*, 1987).

The risk of childhood accidents remains strongly correlated to poverty, and there is a need to make both deprivation and accident prevention a priority for policy makers (Ness *et al.*, 2002), both at local and national level, particularly as injury and death rates are far higher for those in lower socio-economic groups in all types of accidents. The Government-funded Sure Start scheme (Department for Education and Skills (DfES), 2003a) is one such scheme to tackle health inequalities, posed by, among other things, poverty. It was specifically designed to improve the life chances of babies and young children from disadvantaged backgrounds and has a particular target of reducing accident rates. These schemes are based in socially deprived areas thereby targeting and effectively reaching those families most in need (Haynes *et al.*, 2003).

Economics is concerned with the amount of money families have to spend. In Jack's case, his mother is unemployed and living on benefits. She will have to prioritise her outgoings making food and rent more important than safety equipment. Kendrick and Marsh (2001) found that families themselves highlighted low income as an important barrier to providing home safety, a solution for which may be the provision of locally based affordable safety-

**Table 10.2** Socio-economic factors related to injury *(Source: Towner* et al., *2005)*

- Lack of money (ability to buy safety equipment)
- Exposure to hazardous environments inside and outside the home (facilities for safe play; smoking parents; older wiring; lack of garden; small, cramped accommodation)
- Ability of parents/carers to supervise children (single parent families; parents' maturity, awareness and experience; large family size; family illness, such as depression)
- Children's attitudes and behaviour (risk taking)
- Access to information and services

equipment schemes. Although there is sufficient evidence to suggest that socio-economic factors impinge upon children and their risk of sustaining an accident, little consideration is given to the implications of these social gradients in terms of research (Spencer, 2000). For example, are health-education messages appropriately packaged to target the right audience or are they too often geared at middle-class families (Wall, 1998), taking into consideration the language used in health-promotion materials? This should be an important consideration when developing strategies to prevent accidents, if they are to prove effective.

## HOUSING/HOME ENVIRONMENT

The amount of money Jack's mother has will also affect the home she can provide for them to live in, and the environment can subsequently increase the risk of accidents. This can be due to both the physical environment and housing conditions (Harker and Moore, 1996). Within the home there may be the environmental hazards associated with poor housing and overcrowding. Therefore, it is important to take into consideration that accidents happen in places as well as to people. In Jack's case, he is living on the sixth floor. So how does that increase his risk of accidents?

Most deaths and serious injuries to preschool children occur in the home, hence the significance of the housing factor. This can be compounded if the home is in a poor state of repair, which can be for any number of reasons. Furthermore, families may not prioritise safety equipment as essential purchases if they are living on a limited income. Another reason for high levels of accidents within the home can be due to lack of parental supervision. The child, owing to their developmental level, and the parent, owing to their parenting skills, may have a limited awareness of what is unsafe behaviour. Some of these issues have been targeted and tackled by improved safety standards and regulations, for example the redesigning of kettle flexes which are coiled but stretch, which prevents them from overhanging from the worktop, and plastic bags that now have air vents to prevent suffocation.

Jack is at risk of accidents not only inside the home but also outside of it. These dangers can be the result of less safe environments in disadvantaged areas, such as dangerous streets, poor-quality housing and unprotected industrial and building sites (Haynes *et al.*, 2003), water safety with ponds and the risk of falls from high-rise blocks of flats. Reading *et al.* (1999) found that high rates of accidents were concentrated in areas with large local authority housing estates; the risk of an accident is nearly 50 times greater in the most deprived areas compared with the least deprived. Thus, environmental disadvantages increase the risk of accidents to young children (Judge and Benzeval, 1993; Graham, 1994), such as Jack. In order to address this, policy makers need to ensure that some measures target accident prevention in deprived neighbourhoods, by improving the general quality of the social and physical environment, because the increased risk is significantly associated with these areas and not just because poor families live there (Reading *et al.*, 1999).

Lessons may need to be learnt from other countries where, for example, street environments are safer with priority being given to pedestrians and cyclists, such as the Dutch 'woonerfs', rather than just to motor traffic, and supervised play areas with safe environments around housing (McCarthy, 1996), all of which can help to prevent accidents involving children. Importantly, as children grow and develop they construct their landscapes of risk and safety around categories of private, local and public spheres. Although children's opinions are not often sought, Harden's (2000) study explored the ways in which children and parents deal with risk, safety and danger. She found that children described their private sphere of the home in terms of safety and security, yet expressed concerns about their own vulnerability in public life. The local sphere was in relation to the proximity to the home and also associated with familiarity with places and people. These are additional factors that need to be considered when promoting accident-prevention strategies.

---

**Activity**
*Think of a child that you know and make a list of any risks of accidents posed to them inside and outside of the home.*

---

## PARENTAL FACTORS

Parents have a fundamental responsibility towards safeguarding or promoting their child's welfare (DH, 1989); this could be interpreted to include reducing the risk of accidents to their children. They can achieve this by providing a safer home environment, for example through the use of stair gates and cupboard locks, but also by education and the supervision of their children (Harker and Moore, 1996). However, this will be dependent upon their socioeconomic status and their own knowledge base in relation to what constitutes danger to their child. Being able to assess the needs of the child and family is central if activities regarding accident prevention are to be targeted effectively. To do this, they must take into consideration a number of parental issues which can be contributory factors in childhood accidents, such as lone parenthood and parental stress. It is important to avoid adopting a 'blame' approach when working with families: often, the circumstances families find themselves in are beyond the parents' control.

Jack's mother is a single parent, and it has been demonstrated (Roberts and Pless, 1995) that this factor can also increase the risk of accidents. This is because the children of British lone mothers have injury rates that are twice those of children in two-parent families (Roberts and Pless, 1995) and the highest death rates of all socio-economic groups (Judge and Benzeval, 1993). But not only is Jack's mother single – she is 18 years of age.

Maternal age can be a contributory factor as childhood accident rates increase as maternal age decreases (Kendrick and Marsh, 2001). One reason suggested may be the lack of supervision and control over children whose temperament and behaviour lead them into hazardous situations (Reading *et al.*, 1999).

Lack of supervision can be a major contributory factor, as Sharples *et al.* (1990) found in their study. Out of 71 children killed from a fatal head injury while playing; only one had a parent present. Compared to single-adult households, households with four adults had childhood injury rates reduced by 31% and serious injury rates reduced by 42% (Haynes *et al.*, 2003). Hence, Jack is at greater risk, for example if Jack's mother goes into the kitchen there is no one else to watch Jack for her. Often, lone parents have limited resources in terms of social support; this is unfortunate as social support promotes health. It has been recognised that in child rearing the relationship with a partner can be an important source of emotional support and a means of accessing information (Cohen and Syme, 1985). Be aware of the importance of the development of support mechanisms for parents, which allow greater adult supervision of children. This can be through the setting up of groups which enable parents in similar situations to network and befriend other parents, such as Gingerbread groups (<http://www.gingerbread.org.uk>).

Lack of support, divorce, death in the family, chronic illness, homelessness, moving house, unemployment and financial worries are examples of established risk factors for maternal depression, which in turn is a risk factor for childhood injury. A recent study by McLennan and Kotelchuck (2000) found that mothers of toddlers and preschool-aged children with high levels of depressive symptoms were less likely to apply preventive practices, such as using a car seat and/or using electrical plug covers, while Wall (1998) recognised that parental depression and stress play a key part in causes of accidents, as they affect the carer's ability to meet the needs of their children. In Jack's case, there are a number of issues causing his mother concern and raising her levels of anxiety.

One suggestion to help such parents is by providing increased day-care facilities for preschool children, as this would enable parents to enter the workforce and offer a means of increasing their income and their social interaction (Roberts and Pless, 1995), which in turn may reduce accidents by relieving parental stress. Public-funded places for day care for children under 3 years of age are 2% in Britain, compared to 20% in France and 48% in Denmark (Labour Research Department, 1991). However, subsequent governments have introduced a range of policies to address these deficits. Furthermore, the safety of day-care environments, both in the UK and abroad, is regulated, hence ensuring a safe environment for children who may otherwise be exposed to the environmental hazards of living in poverty.

This is important, especially because, as Long *et al.* (2001) found in their research studying the effectiveness of parenting programmes facilitated by health visitors, 25.6% of parents stated that their child's medical problems and accidents were their most stressful experiences, which would increase the levels of stress experienced. This is due to the fact that accidents do not allow parents or children to prepare themselves for the stressful experience of attending hospital, hence anxiety levels are heightened (Hatcher *et al.*, 1993; Brackenbury and Duggan, 1996). Being aware of factors that may cause stress and depression may help when developing appropriate accident-prevention strategies.

Culture or ethnicity is another acknowledged contributory factor in the risk of accidents (Towner *et al.*, 2005). Although little explored, what has been investigated tends to focus on minority ethnic groups. It is important to appreciate and respect that culture has the potential to affect and impinge on all facets of life. For example, child-rearing practices such as those related to supervision, independence and appropriate play activities for children are socially and culturally determined (Soori and Bhopal, 2002); understanding these factors can help understand how the child's ethnicity can impact upon the risk of accidents. A study by Tobin *et al.* (2002) conducted in Leicester found that children from south Asian backgrounds had a 40% lower rate of accident admissions; however, they concluded this may be due to their lower level of participation in physical activities. Adopting a wider approach and recognising the cultural attitudes to safety and child supervision may help understand and acknowledge the impact these may have upon the child's risk of accidents.

## GOVERNMENT POLICY AND ACCIDENT PREVENTION

In order to engage in accident prevention in practice, an understanding of the strategies and policies that have been implemented and which through collaborative practice should result in a reduction in the incidence of child accidents is necessary.

In 1999, the Government set a target in the White Paper *Our Healthier Nation* that accident statistics must be reduced by a fifth by the year 2010. In this paper, it is recognised that accidents are the greatest single threat to life for children and young people. The link between social deprivation and accident was also highlighted and a commitment to narrowing this gap was made. The Government's strategy to ensure improved health was by a collaborative three-way partnership between the State, local communities and individuals.

The cross-Government taskforce report *Preventing Accidental Injury: Priorities for action* (DH, 2002a) emphasises the need to prevent injury to children particularly and leads with the argument that accidents are not inevitable. The taskforce adopted children and young people for priority attention. The report recommends a more united approach to accident prevention across Government and the NHS; efforts are to be directed at priority areas where inequalities have been identified. There is a clear recognition that public health has a key role to play in coordinating prevention and surveillance.

The Government's Green Paper *Every Child Matters* (DfES, 2003b) aims to safeguard children by providing the support they need to be healthy and stay safe, and particular attention is directed to those most vulnerable children and young people who are considered to be at most risk from accidents.

## THE NATIONAL SERVICE FRAMEWORK

The *NSF* (DH and DfES, 2004) presents a 10-year programme intended to stimulate long-term and sustained improvement in children's health. Setting standards for health and social services for children, young people and pregnant women, the *NSF* aims to ensure fair, high-quality and integrated health and social care from pregnancy, right through to adulthood. The *NSF* is divided into three parts: part one contains standards 1–5 and pertains to all children, young people and their parents or carers; part two contains standards 6–10 and pertains to those children who have particular needs; part three addresses the needs and choices of women and their babies before pregnancy through to the first 3 months after birth. Although the *NSF* reiterates and explores a number of the factors discussed above, the following points focus upon accident prevention.

- 'All Primary Care Trusts and local authorities to have in place child and family health promotion programmes which include targeted programmes for vulnerable groups and address national public health priorities – one of which is accident prevention' (DH and DfES, 2004, p. 43).
- 'Primary Care Trusts and local authorities ensure that childhood injuries and accidents are reduced through the development and monitoring of injury prevention strategies that target priority areas where there are marked inequalities. A named lead in each locality develops, co-ordinates and monitors initiatives for tackling injury prevention. This would contribute to the national target to reduce the number of children killed or seriously injured by 2010' (DH and DfES, 2004, p. 50).
- 'Parents with very young children receive advice from home visitors and other family advisers regarding the practical steps to take to protect their children against falls, scalding, burns, drowning, choking and poisoning' (DH and DfES, 2004, p. 50).

- 'Early years settings, schools and local authorities ensure that school-age children are encouraged to participate in safety training schemes run by schools, local authorities or voluntary organisations, such as cycling proficiency, and effective safety training should be provided for those who work with children and young people' (DH and DfES, 2004, p. 50).
- 'Local authorities have clear guidance on the effective use of equipment, such as cycle helmets, child care seats, seat belts, fireguards and stair gates, thermostat controls on hot water taps, and smoke alarms' (DH and DfES, 2004, p. 50).
- 'Primary Care Trusts and local authorities, in partnership with other local agencies, work together to make the local environment safer for children and young people, including undertaking injury surveillance, and sharing data effectively' (DH and DfES, 2004, p. 50).
- 'Schools also have a responsibility to provide information on health related matters such as injury prevention' (DH and DfES, 2004, p. 57).
- 'The information provided locally to parents by health, education and social care agencies includes accident prevention and reducing non-intentional injury, as well as the safe storage of medicines and volatile substances within the home' (DH and DfES, 2004, p. 74).
- 'Schools with support from other agencies support young people in exploring and managing risk and encourage less harmful behaviours through personal, social and health education (PSHE) and citizenship programmes as part of a "whole school approach"' (DH and DfES, 2004, p. 130).
- 'Local authorities reduce injuries to, and deaths of, young people through local initiatives such as action to reduce drowning, and traffic calming and careful siting of public play areas' (DH and DfES, 2004, p. 130).
- 'Serious care reviews are conducted where a child sustains a potentially life-threatening injury' (DH and DfES, 2004, p. 160).

The Government has raised awareness by supporting organisations and campaigns targeting accident prevention in children such as the following.

- Sure Start, working in conjunction with the CAPT to raise awareness of the importance of accident prevention nationally and locally. Booklets entitled 'I'm only a baby, but . . .' have been produced through these organisations to support parents on a one-to-one or group basis in giving guidance on how to keep their baby safe.
- The Foundation for the Study of Infant Death has had significant success in its campaigns related to safe sleeping and the avoidance of parents sharing beds with babies.
- Seasonal safety campaigns targeting high-risk times, such as summer where water-related injuries and cycling injuries occur, can increase awareness by ensuring poster presentations and related leaflets, for example, are displayed in all clinical areas. These resources can be obtained through local health-promotion centres.

- Cycle helmet campaigns have reduced the incidence of serious head injury and can be promoted collaboratively in health and educational communities alike, as can road safety campaigns such as the 'Hedgehog' initiative teaching young children how to cross the road safely.
- Raising awareness of teen road safety has become an essential focus particularly with the 11–14 age group, where boys in particular have been found to be at high risk of serious injury as a result of pedestrian road traffic accidents. The *'Think'* campaign has also been designed to engage young people in considering the catastrophic risks of driving too fast or under the influence of alcohol.

This is a small sample of some of the strategies that are in place to help raise awareness of accident prevention.

## CONCLUSION

The challenges of addressing accident prevention are an ongoing, but vital, area for delivering quality service provision and reducing unnecessary injury and death to children. This chapter has attempted to raise awareness of accident prevention, and how a secure knowledge base of both the developmental stages of childhood and the factors affecting the risk of accidents in childhood will assist with promoting accident prevention in a variety of settings, including the child's own home. By working through the activities provided, it is intended that the reader will continue to develop their knowledge base and practice skills for the future.

## REFERENCES

Bara V (2002) Substances of low toxicity by ingestion. *Emergency Nurse* 10(6), 21–26.

Bates N (2001) Acute poisoning: Bleaches, disinfectants and detergents. *Emergency Nurse* 8(10), 14–19.

Bee H and Boyd D (2000) *The developing child* (9th edn). Harlow: Longman.

Brackenbury C and Duggan H (1996) *Evaluation of the Positive Parenting Project.* London: Hillingdon Health Agency.

CAPT (2005) http://www.capt.org.uk (accessed May 2006).

Cohen S and Syme L (eds) (1985) *Social Support and Health.* New York: Academic Press.

Department for Education and Skills (DfES) (2003a) *Birth to Three Matters: A framework to support children in their earliest years.* London: DfES.

Department for Education and Skills (DfES) (2003b) *Every Child Matters.* Presented to Parliament by the Chief Secretary to the Treasury by Command of Her Majesty, Cm 5860. Norwich: HMSO.

Department of Health (DH) (1989) *The Children Act.* London: HMSO.

Department of Health (1999) *Saving Lives: Our healthier nation white paper and reducing health inequalities.* London: TSO.

Department of Health (DH) (2000) *Framework for the Assessment of Children in Need and their Families.* London: TSO.

Department of Health (DH) (2002a) *Preventing Accidental Injury: Priorities for action.* London: TSO.

Department of Health (DH) (2002b) *Accidents are Not Inevitable: Government sets priorities for action.* London: TSO.

Department of Health and Department for Education and Skills (DH/DfES) (2004) *National Service Framework for Children, Young People and Maternity Services: Core standards.* London: DH/DfES.

Department of Trade and Industry (1999) *Government Consumer Safety Research: Burns and scalds in the home.* London: DTI.

Graham H (1994) The changing financial circumstances of households with children. *Children and Society* 8, 98–113.

Harden J (2000) There's no place like home: The public/private distinction in children's theorizing of risk and safety. *Childhood* 7(1), 43–59.

Hardey M and Crow G (eds) (1991) *Lone Parenthood: Coping with constraints and making opportunities.* Toronto: University of Toronto Press.

Harker P and Moore L (1996) Primary health care action to reduce home accidents: A review. *Health Education Journal* 55(3), 322–331.

Hatcher JW, Powers LL and Richtmeier AJ (1993) Parental anxiety and response to symptoms of minor illness in infants. *Journal of Pediatric Psychology* 18(3), 397–408.

Haynes R, Reading R and Gale S (2003) Household and neighbourhood risks for injury to 5- to 14-year-old children. *Social Science and Medicine* 57(4), 625–636.

Hendry L and Kloep M (1996) Is there life beyond 'flow'? *Proceedings of the 5th Biennial Conference of the EGARA.* University of Liege, May, 1996.

Holt L (1993) The adolescent in accident and emergency. *Nursing Standard* 8(8), 30–34.

Illingworth RS (1991) *The Normal Child.* London: Churchill Livingstone.

Jarman B (1983) Identification of underprivileged areas. *British Medical Journal* 286(6379), 1705–1709.

Judge K and Benzeval M (1993) Health inequalities: New concerns about the children of single mothers. *British Medical Journal* 306(6879), 677–680.

Kendrick D and Marsh P (2001) How useful are sociodemographic characteristics in identifying children at risk of unintentional injury? *Public Health* 115(2), 103–107.

Labour Research Department (1991) *Bargaining Report III.* London: LRD.

Laing GL and Logan S (1999) Patterns of unintentional injury in childhood and their relation to socio-economic factors. *Public Health,* 113(6), 291–294.

Long A, McCarney S, Smyth G, Magorrian N and Dillon A (2001) The effectiveness of parenting programmes facilitated by health visitors. *Journal of Advanced Nursing* 34(5), 611–620.

McCarthy M (1996) Controversy, children and cycle helmets: The case against. *Child: Care, Health and Development* 22(2), 105–111.

McCrea S and Bates N (1999) Acute iron overdose. *Emergency Nurse* 7(5), 18–23.

McLennan JD and Kotelchuck M (2000) Parental prevention practices for young children in the context of maternal depression. *Pediatric* 105(5), 1090–1095.

Ness V, Hoskins R and Robb A (2002) The use of childhood injury surveillance within a general accident and emergency department. *Accident & Emergency Nursing* 10(3), 170–176.

*Oxford English Dictionary* (2005) *Oxford English Dictionary* (3rd edn). Edited by Soanes C and Hawker S. Oxford: Oxford University Press.

Piaget J (1977) *The Development of Thought.* New York: Viking Press.

Pless B (1993) *The Scientific Basis of Injury Prevention: A review of the medical literature.* London: CAPT.

Reading R, Langford IH, Haynes R and Lovett A (1999) Accidents in preschool children: Comparing family and neighbourhood risk factors. *Social Science and Medicine* 48(1999), 321–330.

Roberts I and Pless B (1995) For debate: Social policy as a cause of childhood accidents: The children of lone mothers. *British Medical Journal* 311(7010), 925–928.

Sharples PM, Storey A, Aynsley-Green A and Eyre JA (1990) Causes of fatal childhood accidents involving head injury in Northern region 1979–1986. *British Medical Journal* 301, 1193–1197.

Sheridan MD (1997) *From Birth to Five Years: Children's developmental progress.* London: Routledge.

Siegler RS (2005) *Children's Thinking* (4th edn). Upper Saddle River, NJ: Prentice Hall.

Soori H and Bhopal RS (2002) Parental permission for children's independent outdoor activities: Implications for injury prevention. *European Journal of Public Health* 12(2), 104–109.

Spencer N (2000) Social gradients in child health: Why do they occur and what can paediatricians do about them? *Ambulatory Child Health* 6(3), 191.

Taylor J and Müller D. (1995) *Nursing Adolescents.* London: Blackwell Science.

Tobin MD, Milligan J, Shukla R, Crump B and Burton PR (2002) South Asian ethnicity and risk of childhood accidents: An ecological study at enumeration district level in Leicester. *Journal of Public Health Medicine* 24(4), 313–318.

Towner E (2002) *The Prevention of Childhood Injury: Background paper for the accidental injury task force September 2002.* University of Newcastle Upon Tyne.

Towner E, Dowswell T, Erring G, Burkes M and Towner J (2005) *Injuries in children aged 0–14 years and inequalities.* A report prepared for the Health Development Agency. London: HDA.

Townsend P, Phillimore P and Beattie A (1987) *Health and Deprivation: Inequality and the North.* London: Croom Helm.

United Nations Children's Fund (UNICEF) (2002) *Implementation Handbook for the Convention on the Rights of the Child.* New York: UNICEF.

Wall A (1998) Childhood accidents: A major problem worth tackling. *Professional Care of Mother and Child* 6(3), 200–202.

www.gingerbread.org.uk (accessed May 2006).

www.hassandlass.org.uk (accessed May 2006).

www.sids.org.uk/fsid/babyzone1.htm (accessed May 2006).

# 11 Safeguarding Children

**D. HARRIS AND H. RUSSELL-JOHNSON**

## INTRODUCTION

This chapter will examine the contribution that healthcare workers of all levels can make in the protection of children. Definitions taken from *Working Together to Safeguard Children* (Department of Health (DH), 1999) and discussion of child-protection procedures used in England will be used to demonstrate that all personnel involved in the care of children have a duty to ensure that a child's welfare is maintained (Children Act 2004, see Chapter 12, p. 249). The obligation to safeguard children placed on individuals since the Children Act 2004 can appear daunting; however, what has to be remembered is that the two people who tried hardest to save Victoria Climbié were a childminder and a taxi driver (Laming, 2003).

It is assumed that all children live in supportive households; however, 26 300 children's names were registered with Social Services departments on the Child Protection Register at the end of 2004 in England alone. While this is a slight decrease in numbers on previous years, children still remain vulnerable (DfES, 2005).

The Child Protection Register is a database held by Social Services departments that contains the names of all local children who currently have unresolved protection issues and who require help from more than one support agency, for example Children, Schools and Family departments. Having your name on this list does not offer protection in itself. However, it alerts professionals to the fact that the child and family require ongoing support and it is also a way to ensure that children receive the care that they require (Barker and Hodes, 2004), for example if a health visitor is concerned that a child is not meeting developmental milestones because of poor parental interaction and the carers are refusing to work in partnership with healthcare professionals, following procedures laid down in local safeguarding policies, the child's name may be placed on the Child Protection Register. This means that the child is allocated a key worker and that certain conditions will be given to ensure that the child gets the care he or she needs. If the carers refuse to adhere to the specified criteria, for example attending clinic, further action may result, possibly culminating in the child being fostered or, in extreme cases, adopted.

*Caring for Children and Families.* Edited by I. Peate and L. Whiting
© 2006 John Wiley & Sons Ltd

Statistics indicate that nationally between two and four children each week will die at the hands of their carers as a result of abuse or neglect and many more will suffer long-term emotional problems (Barker and Hodes, 2004). The National Health Service (NHS) employs 1.3 million people (<http://www.doh. gov.uk>). As children form a large proportion of service users, there is every chance that each healthcare professional has been, or will become, involved in some form of safeguarding procedure.

All healthcare workers have a 'duty to protect'. This means that they are obliged to listen to children and act on what they are told. All organisations have a 'duty to cooperate' (Children Act 2004). This means that, even if your care group is not primarily children, you will have to have knowledge of how to support and refer them should a concern over their safety be raised.

Workers who are involved in the care of children will have regular updates in relation to safeguarding policy and procedure. Unfortunately, often all that is remembered from these study days are the scenarios which have been used to enhance the statistics – the protection policies and support systems are often forgotten. This chapter is not intended to replace these study days but to supplement the knowledge gained by highlighting important aspects of child-protection recognition and referral.

## WHY DO CHILDREN NEED PROTECTING?

'Child protection' is the term used by all agencies when there is a suspicion that abuse is taking place. Put in its simplest terms, 'child abuse' is any treatment of a child which is harmful or morally wrong (Munro, 2002). The person inflicting the harm or potential harm is called the 'perpetrator' (Stower, 1999).

The perpetrators of abuse are not necessarily parents or families; they can be anyone that the child has contact with, including other children and healthcare professionals. Over the last 30 years, there have been over 70 high-profile child-protection cases (National Society for the Prevention of Cruelty to Children (NSPCC), 2005). These are the ones that make the headlines, make us stop and think and then carry on with our lives. However, these children are the children that are known about and do not include children who:

- remain silent about the abuse
- are bullied at home or school
- work within the sex trade
- are homeless
- live in abusive relationships
- have parents with mental health problems, substance-abuse or learning-disability issues
- are seeking asylum
- cannot discuss their situation because of a disability
- do not have English as a first language.

It does not follow that children who have been abused will become abusers themselves. However, any form of abuse will be detrimental to certain aspects of a child's development and may affect the child in their adult life.

The United Nations Convention on the Rights of the Child (Article 19, UNCRC, 1989) states that there is an obligation to protect children from all forms of maltreatment perpetrated by parents or others responsible for their care and preventive treatment should be undertaken where required. This implies that all parental actions should take full account of the child's best interest and that when carers fail the State must intervene (Beckett, 2003). However, it also assumes that there is knowledge of abuse taking place. Children may suffer abuse in silence well into adulthood, with some never admitting that the abuse has occurred. This is why carers of children must have an understanding of the safeguarding children policies and procedures for their area of work and have communication skills that are developed well enough to know what a child is trying to say, with or without words. If concerns are raised over the safety of a child, it is essential to discuss these with a senior member of staff before any decision is taken.

## CHILDREN'S PLACE IN SOCIETY

Until the early nineteenth century, children were viewed as the property of their parents. They were expected to earn their keep and life was harsh for some children (NSPCC, 2005). In 1884, the London Society for the Prevention of Cruelty to Children was formed. This later became the National Society for the Prevention of Cruelty to Children. Following this, several changes in law occurred surrounding the safeguarding of children, most of which followed high-profile child-protection cases. The identified problem always appeared to be the same: the failure of the professionals to work together and to listen to the children about what had happened and what they wanted.

The most significant piece of legislation aimed at protecting children was the Children Act (Part 1, 1989, see Chapter 12, p. 245), which states 'the welfare of the child is paramount', that is the child and their wishes must be put first. There is also an expectation that children are usually best looked after by their families. Although the emphasis of the Act was on family rather than parents, the concept of parental responsibility was introduced. The Act advocated that no action in regard to the child should be taken unless it actively benefited the child and that at all times the child's voice should be heard. Despite these innovations, children continued to die at the hands of their carers.

*Working Together to Safeguard Children* (DH, 1999) recognises that agencies need to work together more effectively and use a common language and assessment framework. It identifies what should constitute reasonable parental care and that specific groups of children are more at risk. This was followed by the Children and Adoption Act 2002 and the Sexual Offences Act

2003. However, it was the death of Victoria Climbié that resulted in some of the major changes in the safeguarding of children. The Laming Report (2003) and subsequent green paper *Every Child Matters* (DfES, 2004) highlighted the need for change. This resulted in the Children Act 2004, which pulled together the recommendations from the inquiry into Victoria's death, the Human Rights Act 1998, the Convention on the Rights of the Child 1989 and the Children Act 1989. This has culminated in five clear themes for the protection of children. These are that they should:

• stay safe
• be healthy
• enjoy and achieve
• achieve economic well-being
• make a positive contribution.

*Every Child Matters* (DfES, 2004), therefore, suggests that any strategic approach for the protection of children should consider the following:

• the rights of the child to be protected
• family resources
• education
• support for families in need
• protection of children from abuse.

Since the Children Act 2004, all NHS Trusts are required to ensure that all staff who are likely to have access to children or vulnerable individuals should have the appropriate pre-employment checks, education, updating and super-vision to comply with safeguarding procedures competently. Each Trust must have a designated nurse and doctor who can be contacted in relation to child-protection concerns and who will organise appropriate educational pro-grammes. Their names will appear in the Trust's safeguarding children policy. These criteria are echoed in section 5 of the *National Service Framework for Children* (NSF) core standards (DH and DfES, 2004). This is also discussed in Chapter 12.

## IDENTIFYING ABUSE: DEFINING KEY TERMS

Concerns around the welfare of children can arise in many contexts. Many of the questions asked when a child is considered at risk include the following.

• What is the cause of concern?
• Is there significant harm?
• Is the harm attributable to the care being given?
• What is the severity of the harm, and is it likely to continue?
• Is the parenting good enough?
• What are the consequences of leaving things as they are?

The following sections will aim to clarify the definitions of abuse and harm and equip healthcare workers with the strategies to attempt to answer some of these questions and achieve the best outcomes for children. All the definitions have been drawn from DH (1999) because one of the main drivers for interagency working is the use of a common language and common framework for assessment.

## WHO IS A CHILD IN NEED?

Under the terms of the Children Act 1989, a child in need is one whose vulnerability is such that the child is unlikely to reach or maintain a satisfactory level of health or development, or their health and development will be impaired without the provision of services (s 17(10) Children Act 1989). This is also discussed in Chapter 12.

## WHAT IS SIGNIFICANT HARM?

This concept was originally introduced by the Children Act 1989 (s 47). The Local Authority (Social Services) has a duty to investigate where there is reasonable cause to suspect that a child might, or is likely to, suffer significant harm. This definition was expanded in the Children and Adoption Act 2002 to include the viewing of pornography and domestic violence. Concerns around animal welfare will also heighten awareness around the safety of a child, as research has shown a link between maltreatment of animals and child abuse (Becker and French, 2004).

Guidelines to decision-making are included in DH (2000). If there is a problem in one or more of the component parts, further investigation will take place. Good practice suggests that at all times referrals and investigations should closely involve the child and family; however, there may be occasions when it is not in the child's best interest to inform the carers, for example if sexual abuse is suspected. Therefore, factual, clear and concise documentation is essential to demonstrate all interactions with the family. This will allow all practitioners to have access to the same information and build a cohesive picture of family life.

## IMMEDIATE PROTECTION

If a child is thought to be in immediate need of protection, for example the home circumstances are unsafe or the care provided by a carer with parental responsibility (see Chapter 12) is so inadequate that the child is in danger and needs to be removed to a place of safety, an Emergency Protection Order (EPO) can be sought. This is usually obtained by social workers who have to apply to a magistrate for the order (Children Act 1989, s 44). The EPO lasts eight days and can be extended by another seven days if risk to the child remains. Under an EPO, the Local Authority shares parental responsibility with the carers; this means, for example, that a social worker may give consent for examination or treatment of the child.

The police also have the power to issue Police Protection Orders (PPOs) if they feel that the child needs to be taken to a place of safety, for example if a child is found home alone. This effectively places the child in police protection for 72 hours (Children Act 1989, s 46). Only the police have the statutory right of entry into premises where a child is thought to be at risk.

If the child is not in immediate danger, an Interim Care Order (ICO) can be sought; this also gives Social Services joint parental responsibilities with the carers. However, neither the PPO nor the ICO gives the power to insist on medical treatment if the parents refuse; other orders will have to be sought to address this.

Children subject to the above orders will usually have to be supervised when visited by their carers. The responsibility of the healthcare worker is to accurately document all observed interactions. If a carer attempts to remove the child, you will need to follow your Trust/organisation's protocol for violence and aggression. You cannot prevent a carer leaving with their child, but you must ensure that senior staff, the police and Social Services are notified immediately.

WHAT IS ABUSE?

Abuse is what the child perceives as unacceptable behaviour. This goes beyond the usual childhood anxieties and, if left unresolved, may have a long-term impact on the child's physical and emotional well-being. Abuse can be caused by neglect, inflicting or not preventing harm, not meeting the child's developmental or emotional needs or failure to meet their basic needs, including medical treatment (DH, 1999). The perpetrator can be a friend, family, institution or community. While children are continually told not to talk to strangers, the threat of stranger danger only accounts for 10% of child abuse. Children are more likely to be abused by people that they know (NSPCC, 2005). This was recognised by the Sexual Offences Act 2003 (s 10), which changed the laws on incest to include parental partners. Cases of child abduction are often opportunistic and are rarely planned.

Children may also be abused by other children; bullying is a good example of this. Bullying is a power-based relationship. And yet, currently, it is not recognised under child protection, as it does not necessarily involve the parents. Child-on-child abuse may take many forms, for example the case of James Bulger in 1993. In all cases, the perpetrator is also a victim, but this is often forgotten.

As with other aspects of human nature, there are factors which will aggravate the chances of harm and those which mitigate protection. This will include the child's own coping and adapting mechanisms, support of family and social network, subsequent life events and the response of professional agencies. This is an aspect which is commonly overlooked (DH, 1999).

## CATEGORIES OF ABUSE

Abuse is divided into four categories:

- physical
- emotional
- neglect
- sexual.

Often where one form of abuse occurs so does another; this is because of the behaviours exhibited by the perpetrator. Children can suffer abuse anywhere, including at the hands of people they trust, making it more difficult for them to disclose to others outside the abusive relationship. This gives the perpetrator power and forms the basis of the relationship. Coercion, threats and consequences are common and place an added burden on the child. This is why enhanced observation and communication skills are required to enable the child to disclose their situation.

### Physical abuse

This is seen as a continuum with permanent physical damage and death at one end of the spectrum and minor injuries and bruising that are inflicted deliberately by the carer at the other. This can involve hitting, shaking, throwing, poisoning or otherwise causing physical harm to a child, including fabricating illness. This is where a carer will deliberately induce illness in a child to gain the attention of the medical profession (this is also known as 'fabricated illness by carer' or 'Munchausen's by Proxy' (DH, 2002). If extensive invasive medical tests are carried out to determine diagnosis, the medical profession unknowingly starts to collude in the abuse. There are also cultural aspects to physical abuse; these include female genital mutilation (FGM) and the belief that children can be possessed by spirits.

The main concern related to culture and child protection is that it is not possible to understand all cultural beliefs or rituals. While healthcare workers must respect individual beliefs and uphold them wherever possible, this must not be done to the detriment of a child's welfare or safety. The key is to investigate the behaviour and negotiate that, while this may be the family's belief, there are laws in the UK which demand that we protect children against certain practices. This includes smacking. The Children Act 2004 (s 58) states that reasonable punishment may be used but does not clarify what this means.

Presentation of physical abuse can take many forms, and children can have the most bizarre and unfortunate accidents. There is a great deal of truth in the saying that fact is often stranger than fiction. However, the key to skilled assessment is to view the child and family, and not just the presenting injury, as the complete picture. Paediatric care is based on holistic assessment, but it is often difficult to be objective when it is felt that a child may have been harmed or neglected intentionally.

Certain behaviours from carers and a child's injuries can indicate that the harm the child has suffered may not have been acquired through accidental means; however, there may equally be a perfectly valid reason for the behaviour or injury. That said, further investigation into the situation may be required in the following circumstances:

- delay in seeking medical advice;
- incompatibility of injury to explanation;
- inconsistent story from child and carer;
- multiple injuries at different stages of healing;
- not allowing the child to speak about how the accident occurred;
- and blaming someone else for the injury.

Injuries that show the following patterns should also be questioned:

*Fractures and dislocations*

- spiral fractures, caused by twisting of limbs
- fractures in under 2s or immobile babies
- joint and skull fractures
- rib and collar-bone injuries not associated with trauma
- whiplash not associated with trauma
- multiple fractures of various ages.

*Bruising and lacerations*

- regular pattern of bruising (e.g. finger-tip bruising)
- injury resembles the shape of an object (e.g. cooking utensil, belt buckle)
- restraining marks, especially around wrists and ankles
- bite marks
- bruising at different stages of healing
- inappropriate bruising for type of activity and age (e.g. immobile babies with bruising because they have fallen)
- bruising to genitalia
- abdominal swelling.

*Burns and scalds*

- scalds that go around limbs with no splash marks
- burns and scalds to the soles of the feet
- burns resembling an object (e.g. iron or radiator imprints)
- cigarette or rope burns.

*Chemical*

- unexplained poisoning
- unexplained sudden illness (e.g. sudden onset of seizures or collapse in the absence of underlying illness).

The above list is to provide guidance only; as with all forms of abuse, detection comes from observation, allegation and disclosure. Beware of mistaking an innocent explanation for something more serious or not following up an explanation which does not fit the care that the child appears to have received. The key to understanding is good assessment, documentation and communication – so that disclosures are not lost and false allegations are not made.

Often physical abuse results from outside stressors or a genuine inability to parent because the adult is also vulnerable. Enabling and supporting the carers with the help of other agencies is often all that is needed to enhance their parenting skills.

---

**Activity**
*Do you know what the following are and what they may be mistaken for?*

- *Mongolian blue spots*
- *staphylococcal scalded skin syndrome*
- *Fifths disease*
- *Ringworm*
- *Healing chickenpox scars*

---

**Mongolian blue spots** are bluish discolorations of the skin seen in babies and children with Asian, Afro-Caribbean or Mediterranean colouring; however, they may also be seen on paler skins. They are usually around the buttocks, often in the sacral area, but may also be present on other parts of the body. They can be mistaken for bruises; therefore, if skin discoloration of this type is noted it should be documented so that the carers do not have to repeatedly explain the mark. **Staphylococcal scalded skin syndrome** can be mistaken for scalds; however, clinical investigation will indicate that the child has an infection and the marks may be widespread. **Fifths disease** – *Erythema infectiosum* – is caused by parvovirus B19 and is a viral illness which causes flu-type symptoms and bright red cheeks resembling marks left by a slap. **Ringworm** and **healing chickenpox scars** can be mistaken for cigarette burns.

## Emotional abuse

The persistent failure to meet a child's emotional needs by providing love, guidance and a sense of self-worth can cause adverse effects on the child's emotional development. This may be permanent and lead to mental health and behavioural issues in adult years, which may also include the inability to parent their children in the future. This form of abuse may be especially damaging during infancy, when attachment bonds are being made with significant carers and can affect the child's ability to interact with others (DH, 1999). The inability to support a child's emotional needs may also be seen in families where there are issues around mental health, substance abuse or special-educational needs because of the carer's own vulnerabilities.

The detection of this form of abuse is highly dependent on documentation, as a picture of the family will need to be built over a period of time. Some of the behaviours exhibited may include:

- erosion of the child's self-esteem, by telling them they are worthless, unloved, inadequate or have limited value;
- inappropriate expectations for age, causing feelings of intimidation or fear (e.g. expecting a child to be totally responsible for younger siblings);
- allowing the child to be exploited or corrupted (e.g. exceptionally gifted children being expected to study or practise at levels which exclude the company of their peers);
- failing to meet the child's emotional needs by withdrawing love as a punishment, inability to give emotional warmth, little physical contact with the child, limited eye contact, ignoring the child's attempts at communication;
- overprotection (e.g. not allowing the child to play outside with friends because of an unrealistic fear of stranger danger);
- failure of carer to take action when involved in an abusive relationship (e.g. domestic violence).

Children who are not having their emotional needs met may exhibit many behaviours, which are dependent on their age. These may include:

- abnormally passive/lethargic behaviour
- attention-seeking behaviour
- delayed development in all areas
- nervous behaviour (e.g. eating disorders, bedwetting)
- tantrums (any attention is better than none, even if it is negative)
- low self-esteem
- inability to interact with others
- lack of age-specific imaginary play
- failure to thrive (however, it is essential that medical reasons are excluded as certain medical conditions may also present these features).

While this form of abuse is very difficult to detect on its own, it is often apparent in all the other types of child harm, as withdrawal of attention and affection are used to make the child feel they are responsible for the harm inflicted on them.

## Neglect

This is the most common form of child maltreatment; 50% of children on Child Protection Register have their name in this category (Barker and Hodes, 2004). It is often a major factor in child deaths and is highly dependent on the carer's ability to meet the child's fundamental needs. Therefore, if there are concerns around learning disability, mental health, substance abuse, domestic violence or poverty, there may be unintentional neglect (Beckett, 2003). Neglect is described as persistent or wilful failure to meet a child's physical or psychological needs, resulting in serious impairment to the child's health or development. It may involve elements of physical and emotional abuse, for example failing to provide adequate food, shelter, clothing or education, failing to protect from harm or danger and failure to ensure access to adequate medical attention (DH, 1999).

Physical signs and symptoms may include:

- poor physical growth, sparse hair;
- failure to thrive or extreme obesity;
- poor hygiene, especially teeth and nappy area;
- inappropriate clothing, shelter, food;
- poor health care (e.g. untreated infections, poor immunisation status);
- behavioural problems;
- frequent injuries and delay in seeking medical advice;
- persistently left without supervision;
- extreme cases of neglect may lead to the child's death.

## Sexual abuse

This involves a power-based relationship where the perpetrator has complete control over the child. The child is powerless within the relationship and therefore may also be at risk from other abusers. Often this form of abuse is perpetrated by an individual that the child knows well (a family member, teacher, another child or activity leader). The secrecy, helplessness and belief that it is their fault makes disclosure difficult, and the child will often retract their statement because of the persuasive behaviours used by the perpetrator. This is why if this form of abuse is suspected it must be discussed with a senior member of staff to decide on the course of action to be taken and not with the parents.

Sexual abuse involves forcing or coercing (grooming) a child into sexual activities, whether the child is aware or not, with or without their consent. Activities may include penetrative and non-penetrative acts or encouraging the child to behave in sexually inappropriate ways. This also includes the viewing or taking part in pornography singularly, as a group or via the Internet and engaging in prostitution. The longer the abuse has been occurring, the more traumatised the child will be; this is because of the conditioning tactics that the perpetrator will have employed and the position that they hold in the child's life. The child's ability to cope with the long-term impact will depend on the support that can be given by a non-abusing adult (DH, 1999).

Behaviour that may indicate that sexual abuse is taking place includes:

- sexually transmitted infections, genital warts, unexplained vaginal or penile discharge, bleeding or bruising from genital or anal area;
- inappropriate or sexually explicit play, with knowledge greater than expected for child's age;
- sudden onset of soiling or bed wetting;
- sleeping/eating disorders;
- recurrent abdominal pain or headaches;
- social withdrawal/restlessness;
- self-destructive behaviours (e.g. self-harm, seizures, faints).

In order to safeguard children, communication must be at the level of their understanding. To facilitate this, the health professional must possess a basic understanding of childhood development. The following case study will demonstrate the importance of understanding normal development within the context of child protection.

---

**Activity**

*Casey is 4 years old and has been admitted to the children's ward because she is experiencing pain on passing urine. On examination, her vulval area is found to be very red and inflamed, with minor lacerations. There are also several superficial scratches over her arms. All Casey will say is 'I want to be like Mummy!' and gets upset when you try to communicate with her. Casey's mother can give no explanation for her behaviour or injuries. The Registrar has requested Casey's admission as he is concerned that as no one can provide an explanation for the injuries Casey may have experienced sexual abuse.*

*Later that day when Casey is being bathed, it is noticed that she appears to be performing an activity which resembles masturbation. When she is asked what she is doing, she replies, 'This is softer than Mummy's.' She goes on to explain that Mummy says she mustn't use her sponge, but she does when mummy is not looking.*

*You discuss this with a more senior member of staff who suggests that the mother is asked to bring her sponges in from home. When this is explained to the mother, she laughs, exclaiming that she had been wondering why her exfoliation sponge had kept moving. When the sponges are lined up at bath time, Casey chooses the exfoliation sponge and commences to rub it vigorously all over her body!*

The example above is a clear case that children do not often have the words to describe what is happening to them, or why they are behaving in a particular way. Copying observed behaviour and exploring their bodies is a natural part of growing up. Casey wanted to be like her mummy, so she mimicked the use of the sponge over her body. She also discovered that it was pleasurable to rub the sponge around her vulval area. This is a natural part of exploration and development, but Casey did not have the language to describe this.

Therefore, practitioners who work with children have to be able to communicate at the level of the child's understanding. This is especially true of children with a disability and children whose first language is not English, as it is important to build a picture of the child's life. A fundamental understanding of child development is necessary, and this can be acquired from further reading. Table 11.1 is designed to give some key points of indicative behaviour when observing children who may have been involved in abuse.

Table 11.1 is not a definitive list but an example that children can be affected by abuse in different ways at different ages. However, parental noncompliance with medical treatment at any age must be investigated as this may indicate neglect.

## SUSPICION OF ABUSE

As can be seen from Table 11.1, children who are in need of protection often do not initially appear to be any different from other children of their age. Often suspicion of abuse is raised by a comment or behaviour that appears out of context. This may manifest in an extreme reaction to a routine procedure. To a child who does not understand that not every one treats them the same as the perpetrator of their abuse, the world is a frightening place, but any child can be afraid of unfamiliar surroundings; therefore, as with everything, common sense must prevail. Take care not to judge a child's care by your personal standards: just because children are parented differently from your experience, does not mean that that parenting style is wrong. Child protection is not a stick that parents can be beaten with, but a range of strategies that can move just-good-enough parenting along a continuum to an acceptable standard and enhance the child's quality of life.

---

**Activity**
*Think back to the time you have either had an argument with a close friend or had to tell your child off in public. Would the communication have been the same if you had been at home?*

---

All individuals have a public and private self, and, when they are in public, individuals like to appear in control. Healthcare workers often have a unique

**Table 11.1** Stages of development and indicative behaviour
*(Source: South West Thames Health Authority, 1995)*

| Age (years) | Normal development | Impaired development | Behavioural indicators | Parenting characteristics |
|---|---|---|---|---|
| Birth –1 | Rapid time of growth and muscular control. Social language begins to develop. Significant attachment and trust with others. | Poor muscle control. Failure to thrive. Does not interact with others. Insecure, does not trust carers to come back. Does not reach developmental milestones. | Does not interact with environment. Poor muscle control. Failure to meet developmental milestones. Cries excessively. Lack of social smile. | Unrealistic expectations for child. This can be exhibited by rejecting, isolating or impassive/apathetic behaviour. The parent may place their needs before the child's. |
| 1–3 | Expect others to see world from their point of view. Shows frustration when adults cannot. Motor skills rapidly expand. Child starts to explore world using primary carer as base. If this is not present, the child will have difficulty interacting with others. Parallel play. Starts to notice that all children are not the same. | Poor physical development. Failure to meet milestones. Fearful of new adults. Extreme temper tantrums or poor control of behaviour. Acting out observed. Aggressive behaviour. Apprehension when hearing others cry. Sexually explicit behaviour. | If child has witnessed or been part of a traumatic event, behaviour may start to regress. This may result in clingy and dependent behaviours. They may be incredibly independent, i.e. trying to parent themselves or have extreme temper tantrums or attention-seeking behaviours. Sexual play may be evident. There may be use of vocabulary outside the normal for their age range. Unusual fearfulness. Frozen watchfulness. | All of the above behaviours, but the child is now more aware of being rejected or isolated. There may be unrealistic demands placed on the child, with no boundaries for behaviour. |
| 3–6 | Hungry for information ('Why?') Rapid growth of imaginative play. Rapid expansion of gross motor skills. Starts to enjoy the company of others of a similar age rather than adults. Greater | Lack of interest in surrounding environment. Delayed language and social skills. Poor motor skills. Poor self-esteem, seeing themselves as naughty or unable to be loved. | Frozen watchfulness. May try and precipitate a telling-off to get it over and done with. Guilt at their inability to protect younger siblings or parents. Sleep disturbances. Behavioural problems. Bullying. Aggressive behaviours to self, others, animals. Eating disorders. | All of the above behaviours; however, parental behaviour is specifically directed at the child and may include rejecting, isolating or ignoring the child. Terrorising, sadistic or impassive towards things that the child cares for. |

**Table 11.1** *Continued*

| Age (years) | Normal development | Impaired development | Behavioural indicators | Parenting characteristics |
|---|---|---|---|---|
| | independence: can feed and dress self. Gets frustrated when cannot master new skill. Starts to develop mature sense of right from wrong. | Sexually explicit behaviour or knowledge beyond their years. Bed wetting, soiling. | | Inappropriate demands with unrealistic expectations. Constantly changing boundaries. |
| 6–10 | Beginnings of moral reasoning. Peers becoming more important than parents. Begin to develop a sense of permanence, i.e. a sense of time, space and order. Conscience beginning to develop. | Lack of control. Bullying. Inability to form friendships. Poor concentration. Poor academic performance. Night terrors. Increased reliability on fantasy, yet lacks imagination. Sexually explicit language or behaviour. Poor self-esteem. | Disruptive behaviour, demonstrating behaviours they have observed. Attention seeking. Truanting. Aggressive or withdrawn behaviour. Regression. Bed wetting, soiling. Lack of fear at frightening events. Indiscriminate friendliness and displays of affection. Self-stimulatory behaviour such as rocking or thumb sucking. Sudden onset of phobias. Personality change. Eating disorders. | All of the above but there are also greater elements of control. |
| 10–16 | Growing sense of self. Onset of puberty, strong emotional and sexual feelings. Need to assert independence. Questioning of adult values. Need to experiment. Some rights of passage to adulthood, e.g. arranged marriages and Bar Mitzvah. | Insecurity. Low self-esteem. Intense emotions and identity confusion. The inability to sustain relationships. | Self-destructive or risk-taking behaviours, e.g. drinking, drug taking, violence/ aggression. Self-harm. Constant challenge to authority. Truanting. Inappropriate attention seeking, i.e. sexually provocative behaviour or stealing. Eating disorders. Attention seeking, e.g. shop lifting, vandalism. Superficial friendships. | All of the above with heavy emphasis on the lack of worth that the child has now or in the future. |

insight into private parenting. But when a child is subjected to abusive behaviour in public, when restraint is usually exercised, what will happen when no one is around? If a child is looking frightened, it may be because the term 'Wait till I get you home!' has fearful connotations. If the carers can make staff feel intimidated, think how this may be making the child feel.

The suspicion that the child may be being abused requires health carers to think the unthinkable (Beckett, 2003). There is a broad assumption that healthcare workers are educated for this role and are not affected by it, but there is nothing that can prepare an individual for the strength of their emotions and there is no formula that can tell you how to act in the immediate situation. Often, when abuse is suspected, we try to rationalise and normalise it, by trying to place what we are unsure of into frameworks which do not exist, for example the fact that Victoria Climbié stood to attention when greeting her aunt was put down to culture by the nurses and not questioned (Laming, 2003). Healthcare workers are not expected to be experts in all cultures and religions, but they are expected to use common sense and seek clarification about cultural norms.

## WHAT TO DO ONCE ABUSE IS SUSPECTED

The most important factor is to seek help from a more senior member of staff. There is no option to do nothing. However, there appear to be several factors which influence whether concerns are discussed or not. The major influence seems to be the relationship that we have with the family of the child and also the support that we perceive we will get if we voice our concerns. Relationships with long-term patients appear to cause the most problems as we can start to make excuses for the behaviour. This is known as collusion (Powell, 1997) and may result in:

- becoming part of manipulating behaviour
- confrontation avoidance
- collusion with other professionals
- participation in non-referral
- loss of objectivity.

This is very similar to what happens in 'fabricated illness by carer': the professionals harm the child by inactivity and unnecessary investigations because of the information that is given to them by the carer. Therefore, the relationship between the healthcare worker and the family needs to be established within very tight boundaries. This needs to be done in an empathetic and compassionate manner, rather than befriending families within a more social type of relationship (Robertshaw and Smith, 2004). This can be achieved by following established policies and procedures. These allow the healthcare worker to be confident that their concern will be taken seriously, the child will be protected and they will both be supported.

## WHAT IS A DISCLOSURE?

This is sharing the child's experience and can happen in a variety of ways and will usually include:

- observation
- allegation
- describing experiences.

It is often not by accident that a child will choose to disclose to a junior health-care worker. If you consider the situation through the child's eyes, they may choose to ask for help from a person who works closely with them, whom they do not associate with authority and whom they trust. It is a fallacy that children will ask to share a secret; more often than not there will be a cryptic question to test your response or see if they can trust you, for example, 'Bad things happen to bad children, don't they?' If they do feel confident enough to share their problem, never promise to keep their secret, as you have to share the information to protect them and by betraying their trust you are also abusing them.

## HOW TO DEAL WITH A DISCLOSURE

The most important thing to do is to tell the child how brave they have been and that the situation is not their fault. Explain to them that together you will find a solution to the problem, but you will have to ask others to help you do this and this will involve telling their story to more senior members of staff. The most important thing is that the child still feels they have some form of control over the situation. This is obviously dependent on age. Part 1 of the Children Act (1989) states that the child's welfare is paramount and as a result information must be shared. Once this is done, the incident should be discussed with a senior member of staff and their advice sought. They will also help with documenting the incident, as some of the records may be used to help protect the child in either child-protection or court proceedings. Records need to be:

- clear
- concise
- factual
- dated
- signed.

The disclosure must not be discussed with the child's carers. Although it is best practice to discuss all concerns around children with the family, there are some situations when this may put the child at risk. Discussion with the carers is left to senior staff who will base the information given on the seriousness of the alleged abuse. Where multidisciplinary notes are used at the bedside, senior staff will advise where to document the record of events.

Often abuse is not disclosed but is a culmination of observed events. These observations need to be discussed, just like a disclosure, because clarification for the basis of concern needs to be sought. Your concerns and record of events need to be documented so a picture can be built of the relationship between the child and their carers.

Sometimes, no event is observed, it is just a feeling or overhearing a throw-away comment; again, these all need to be discussed with a senior member of staff to ensure the opinion is objective. Subjectivity plays a very important part in the safeguarding of children: while taking no action is not an option, there are occasions when, following a discussion of events with a senior member of staff, there will be a decision not to refer the child to other professionals. Discuss your anxieties with the member of staff and try to clarify why they do not share your views. If it is because they are unsure of what to do, refer to your local safeguarding children procedures. Also the member of staff may be aware of issues within the family that are not immediately evident to you. In all case, you should document the discussions and their outcome to ensure that you comply with the Children Act 2004. You cannot be responsible for the actions of others, but you must be responsible for your own. The points below may help clarify why sometimes it is easier than at other times to gain support for a child (Powell, 1997).

**What may help with a referral?**

- Access to named, designated professionals
- Clear child-protection procedures
- Personal experience of child maltreatment
- Age of child, type or history of abuse
- Feeling able to share concerns with the family
- Supportive seniors.

**What may hinder a referral?**

- Professional hierarchy and closed systems of working
- Lack of training/updates and professional-development opportunities
- Uncertainty about confidentiality and information sharing
- Lack of confidence in child-protection procedures
- Concerns around personal safety
- A belief in corporal punishment
- Focusing on the vulnerable adult rather than the child
- Concern about losing the therapeutic relationship.

Once you have been involved with any form of child-protection work, you need to discuss your thoughts and feelings with a senior member of staff. This will allow you to reflect and learn from the incident. Many individuals are concerned that the issues surrounding reporting and child-protection work will interfere with the professional relationship; this is especially true in community and school situations, where there may be a longstanding relationship with the family. Healthcare workers are frequently in the best position to help in this situation as they can often identify the crisis point and discuss this with the carers. Good communication is the key. For most forms of abuse, the family should be made aware of the growing concerns around the care of their child so that they can work with healthcare workers to improve their parenting skills. It must be remembered that harm may not always be attributable to poor parenting only. Often external factors may be involved, for example extreme poverty or abuse from outside the family. To ensure sensitivity, try to treat those involved as you would wish to be treated yourself, as often the situation that families find themselves in is part of a wider context of issues over which they have no control.

There may be occasions when it is not possible for the healthcare worker to continue working with the family because of safety issues. These situations need to be resolved on an individual basis in accordance with their Trust's policies. All of the relevant professional bodies concerned with a child-protection issue will wish to support staff directly involved in a child safeguarding situation. This is to enable personal learning to take place, and can take the form of supervision, debriefing meetings or team reflection.

## WHAT IS INTERAGENCY WORKING?

Any action to safeguard children will involve more than one professional group. This is because one of the key principles of the Children Act 2004 is that all relevant agencies work in collaboration to ensure that the jigsaw is pieced together accurately. Based on this information and the sharing of information, an action plan can be written: failure to work together will not provide protection for the child. Following an information-gathering exercise, an initial child-protection meeting will be held. This is an assessment meeting, from this it will be decided whether to follow the child through Section 17 proceedings 'Child in Need' (Children Act 1989, s 17), that is a child who is not in need of protection but in need of support and services, for example a child who has a chronic illness and is unlikely to achieve a reasonable standard of health without the input of a wide range of support services. Alternatively, if the child is in need of protection, the Children, Schools and Families Service have a duty to investigate (Children Act 1989, s 47). The routes that are taken have been clearly laid out in DH (2003) and are also incorporated into local safeguarding children procedures.

Following investigation, a case conference may be held. This is the forum for the sharing of information about individual cases. The initial conference brings together family members and professionals from organisations concerned with child care and protection to share and evaluate information gathered during the investigation. This enables the panel to make decisions about the levels of risk to the child and decide on the need for registration and make plans for the future (DH, 1999).

The main aims of the meeting are to:

- focus on the child and family
- involve the child and family
- listen to the views of others
- share information and assess risk
- make decisions based on the best interest of the child.

If you have been involved in the child's care, you may be asked to attend one of these conferences. However, a senior member of staff will always attend with you. Another inquiry that you may be involved in is when a serious child-protection issue occurs or a child dies while in Local Authority care. There is a review of all the services to determine if any alternative action could have prevented the incident or changes in practice are required. This is known as a 'Chapter 8 Review', as the criteria which it follows come from Chapter 8 of *Working Together to Safeguard Children* (DH, 1999). Although this is a fact-finding and learning exercise, it can be a very stressful experience for all involved. This is why the importance of good documentation and communication skills cannot be emphasised strongly enough.


## CONCLUSION

It is clear that all healthcare workers have a major role to play in the protection of children. The skills involved in the identification of vulnerable children can be incorporated into all areas of private and professional life and may often move outside the boundaries of parenting skills to include wider issues, for example poverty or bullying. The responsibility of safeguarding children is not confined to the work area; sometimes members of staff have issues within their personal life. If you are concerned about a child outside the working environment, the NSPCC, Child Line or Parent Line can be contacted.

There are now many organisations for children that can facilitate disclosure of abuse and will offer support once they have done so. There are also organisations which will help survivors of abuse. These can be accessed through the Occupational Health department or your liaison health visitor. Child abuse thrives on secrecy; therefore, the more open your workplace can be, by displaying help organisations, parenting support classes and domestic violence help lines, the more empowered and educated children and carers can become.

## REFERENCES

Barker J and Hodes D (2004) *The Child in Mind. A child protection handbook*. London: Routledge.

Becker F and French L (2004) Making the links: Child abuse, animal cruelty and domestic violence. *Child Abuse Review* 13(6), 399–414.

Beckett C (2003) *Child Protection. An introduction*. London: SAGE.

Children Act (2004) London: TSO.

Department for Education and Skills (DfES) (2004) *Every Child Matters: Next steps*. London: TSO.

Department for Education and Skills (DfES) (2005) *Statistics of Education: Referrals, assessments and children and young people on Child Protection Registers: year ending 2004*. London: TSO.

Department of Health (DH) (1999) *Working Together to Safeguard Children*. London: DH.

Department of Health (DH) (2000) *Framework for the Assessment of Children in Need and their Families*. London: DH.

Department of Health (DH) (2002) *Safeguarding Children in Whom Illness is Fabricated or Induced*. London: DH.

Department of Health (DH) (2003) *What to Do If You Are Worried a Child Is Being Abused: Children's services guidance*. London: DH.

Department of Health and Department for Education and Skills (DH/DfES) (2004) *National Service Framework for Children and Young People*. London: DH/DfES.

Laming WH (2003) *The Victoria Climbié Inquiry*. Report of an inquiry by Lord Laming. London: TSO.

Munro M (2002) *Effective Child Protection*. London: SAGE.

National Society for the Prevention of Cruelty to Children (NSPCC) (2005) <http://www.nspcc.org.uk> (accessed May 2006).

Powell C (1997) Child protection: The crucial role of the children's nurse. *Paediatric Nursing* 9(9), 13–16.

Robertshaw M and Smith J (2004) Concerned about confidentiality? *Paediatric Nursing* 16(5), 36–38.

South West Thames Health Authority (1995) *Focus on Risk: An aid to decision making at case conferences*. SWTAH: NHS Executive.

Stower S (1999) Principles and practice of child protection. *Paediatric Nursing* 11(7), 35–41.

United Nations Convention on the Rights of the Child (UNCRC) (1989) United Nations General Assembly Document A/RES/44/25.

# 12 Legal Concerns

## H. RUSSELL-JOHNSON AND D. HARRIS

## INTRODUCTION

This chapter considers English law. There are slight variations in Wales, Scotland and Northern Ireland, but the principles are common to all countries of the United Kingdom (UK). The term 'duty of care' is discussed. The term 'child' is defined in legal terms and key law relating to children and health care is outlined briefly. Confidentiality and information sharing are explored in relation to government guidelines. The difference between common law and statute law is discussed in relation to children's consent and refusal. The links between ethics and law are identified, and the four major ethical principles are outlined and related to the care of the child. Finally, human rights and children's rights are discussed in relation to the care of children and young people in children's health services.

## DUTY OF CARE

A duty of care exists if the actions or inactions of an individual are likely to harm someone else. Anyone who may be affected by our actions becomes our neighbour in legal terms. The duty of care is particularly relevant when one is placed in a position of trust and responsibility when caring for others.

Dimond (2005) describes the original case of *Donoghue* v. *Stevenson*, heard in 1932, that highlighted duty of care. A person who bought a bottle of ginger beer found the decomposing remains of a snail when halfway through the bottle and sued the manufacturer arguing that a duty of care was owed by the manufacturer to the consumer. The judge agreed that you must take reasonable care to avoid acts or omissions that may harm your neighbour. A duty of care, therefore, automatically exists as part of the role of carer. It is important, therefore, to know the limits of what you have been trained to do, what you are capable of doing and what you are allowed to do.

*Caring for Children and Families.* Edited by I. Peate and L. Whiting
© 2006 John Wiley & Sons Ltd

## WHAT IS A CHILD?

In English law, a person is a minor or a child until their eighteenth birthday, when the age of majority is achieved. Reaching the age of majority allows a person to vote. This definition is supported by Article 1 of the United Nations Convention on the Rights of the Child (UNCRC, 1989). Children of different ages are often known by different terms. For example, babies under 4 weeks old are called 'neonates'. Other words are 'infant', 'toddler', 'preschool child', 'school-child', 'teenager', 'young person' and 'adolescent'. These terms are not clearly defined, and there is no common agreement about the ages to which they refer. Particularly difficult is the definition of 'adolescence', but for the purposes of this text it is useful to think of adolescents as being of secondary-school age. Whatever term is used, anyone under 18 years is a child where the law is concerned. It is important to differentiate between 'adolescence', which refers to a developmental stage or an age range (for example 12–18 years), and the 'adolescent', a young person within that age range.

## WELFARE VERSUS RIGHTS IN ENGLISH LAW

The concept of rights has been part of civilised life for thousands of years (Wilkinson and Caulfield, 2000). Rights define the relationship between the Government, or authority, and citizens. The international recognition of human rights stemmed from the establishment of the United Nations at the end of the Second World War in 1945. This followed the horrors and the atrocities of war and enabled individual freedom, dignity and justice to become increasingly important in all aspects of life. Health law is becoming increasingly rights based. Children's law, however, has been strongly rooted in welfare (what is good for children) since the end of the nineteenth century and, historically, the State has taken responsibility for the welfare of its children under the ancient doctrine of *parens patriae*, or 'the parent of the country' (Archard, 1993). This doctrine is still used today where judges, acting for the State, overrule the wishes of children to refuse medical treatment. The conflict between rights and welfare is clearly seen in issues of consent and confidentiality.

## WHAT IS LAW?

Law consists of the rules of the State. English law comes from two main sources. The first is statute law. A statute is an Act of Parliament, a law passed by the Houses of Parliament. Parliament can also empower other bodies to pass Statutory Instruments, which have equal power. Some legislation relating to health professionals is made this way. Acts of Parliament and Statutory

Instruments are both statutory sources and as such take precedence over other laws (Dimond, 2005).

The second source is common law, also known as judge made law or case law. Common law is made by the decisions of judges in specific cases. These are often interpretations of statute law and follow a recognised order of precedence. Judges are bound by the outcome of a similar case if, first, it is relevant and, secondly, the judgment was made in a higher court. The relationship of statute law and common law is explored later in relation to children and consent to treatment.

Common law relates only to the way in which the law developed; it has nothing to do with the term 'common law husband' or 'common law wife' used to describe unmarried partners who live together, see 'Parental responsibility' p. 246, below.

## CIVIL AND CRIMINAL LAW

The difference between criminal and civil law lies in how the wrongdoing is managed by the judicial system.

> a breach of the criminal law can be followed by prosecution in the criminal courts, whereas liability in civil law is actionable in the civil courts and may or may not be a crime. (Dimond, 2005, p. 11)

The courts and the penalties are different. A crime occurs when an Act of Parliament is broken, for example theft, common assault or death by dangerous driving. The case is heard by a criminal court which may impose fines, driving bans, community service penalties or imprisonment. A civil offence is a wrong against another person that may or may not involve the breaking of an Act of Parliament. Civil courts hear civil cases, such as libel, and can award damages against a person if they have committed a civil wrong. Civil actions possible in health care include negligence, trespass to the person (see 'Consent', p. 253, below), breach of contract and breach of a statutory duty.

## IMPORTANT LAW IN RELATION TO THE HEALTH CARE OF CHILDREN

### Children Act 1989

The Children Act 1989 came into force in 1991. It is a large piece of legislation that completely revised the relationship between the law, the State and the family. Sections important in the health care of children are detailed below.

*Section 1(1): The welfare of the child*   This states that the welfare of the child is paramount. It is the first time in English law that such a powerful statement has been made. It underlines the welfare (best interests) approach of the law.

*Section 1(3):Welfare checklist*   This identifies what must be taken into account when making decisions about children. The words of the Act relate to decisions reached by a court, but are equally applicable to any decision about children. These include:

- the ascertainable wishes and feelings of the child concerned (considered in the light of their age and understanding);
- the child's physical, emotional and educational needs;
- the likely effect on them of any change in their circumstances;
- their age, sex, background and any characteristics of theirs which are relevant;
- any harm which the child has suffered or is at risk of suffering;
- how capable each of the child's parents, and any other relevant person, is of meeting the child's needs.

*Sections 2–4: Parental responsibility*   This abolished the rule of law that the father is the natural guardian of his legitimate child. The emphasis on parental rights gave way to a focus on the responsibilities of the parents in bringing up their child. Parental responsibility is defined as 'all the rights, duties, powers, responsibilities and authority which by law a parent of a child has in relation to the child and his property'. The details of these are not set out in statute law, but it is generally agreed that these are the things that society expects a parent to do (Hendrick, 1993). These include:

- the provision of a home
- meeting the child's physical and emotional needs
- naming the child
- providing discipline
- providing a religious upbringing
- education
- health care and consent to medical treatment
- parental consent for the marriage of a child over 16 but under 18
- responsibility for transport
- obtaining a passport.

A parent who does not have parental responsibility still has a statutory duty to maintain the child (pay maintenance) and has rights in relation to the child's property in the event of the child's death. The Adoption and Children Act 2002 altered some aspects of parental responsibility (see 'Adoption and Children Act 2002', p. 249, below).

*Who has parental responsibility under the Children Act 1989?*

- A mother has automatic parental responsibility for her child.
- Where the parents were married at the time of the child's birth, both parents share parental responsibility.

- Where more than one person has parental responsibility, each of them may act alone. This means that consent for treatment is only required from one parent.
- After divorce, both parents retain parental responsibility for their child in equal measures.
- A person with a Residence Order (see 'Section 8: Orders', p. 248, below).

### Obtaining parental responsibility

An unmarried father may obtain parental responsibility by:

- making a parental responsibility agreement with the mother and having it recorded formally using an official form and registering the agreement with the Family Court. Forms and accompanying instructions are available from <http://www.hmcourts-service.gov.uk>. This parental responsibility agreement is binding and cannot be undone;
- obtaining a Parental Responsibility Order from the court;
- marrying the mother.

### Others may obtain parental responsibility

This can include grandparents and other family members. The Act identifies who may apply for this, how and under what circumstances.

- The Local Authority may obtain parental responsibility in order to safeguard the child. The child protection orders that allow this are detailed in Chapter 11. Where this happens, the parents retain their parental responsibility but may not exercise it for the duration of the order. The Local Authority, usually in the form of a senior social worker, is the only person who may give valid consent to investigation or treatment of a child under such an order. Consent for photographs or a skeletal survey, for example, will be sought from the social worker, not the parents.
- A person with parental responsibility may arrange for all or some of it to be met by someone acting on their behalf. This transfer of parental responsibility must be in written form. Some examples are:
  - consent for urgent medical treatment on a school trip or cubs' camp is usually handed over to a teacher or Arkela by the person with parental responsibility signing a form to that effect;
  - boarding schools may take on a broader range of parental responsibility duties while the child is in their care;
  - a head teacher may have term-time parental responsibility for a large number of children, particularly where the parents are living abroad;
  - parents may also arrange for parental responsibility to be met by grandparents (e.g. where the child lives with them during school holidays or while the parents are away on a business trip).

*Sections 5–6: Guardianship*    A parent may appoint another person to be the child's guardian in the event of their death. This must be done in a will to be valid. However, such an appointment is not absolute and a guardian may also be appointed by the court. Formally appointed guardians have parental responsibility.

## Section 8: Orders

*These define how parental responsibility may be exercised*    There are four orders the court can make in relation to parental responsibility where there is serious disagreement, but they can only normally be made in respect of a child under 16. The courts will not make any order unless it is better for the child that one is made. This means that the order is made for the benefit of the child, not the parents. The aim of this is to reduce court delays to a minimum. Parents are expected to negotiate agreement in the majority of cases, and the law is used only as a last resort.

- A Contact Order means that the person the child lives with is required to enable the child to have contact with the person named in the order. This is child centred, providing the child with contact, rather than granting contact rights to the adult (e.g. the child may have contact with their grandparent, not the grandparent may have contact with the child).
- A Prohibited Steps Order means that the person with parental responsibility must obtain consent from the court before taking a step, named in the order, which would normally be a part of meeting the parental responsibility. This could be taking the child out of the country.
- A Residence Order states with whom the child is to live. The person or persons named in this order have parental responsibility, but there are some restrictions relating to adoption and guardianship (section 12). You may see this with children in foster care who have reached Local Authority care through a Residence Order. Foster carers know for which children they have parental responsibility; it is part of their education as foster parents. The Residence Order is the only section 8 order that can be made for a child in the care of the Local Authority (section 9). A birth father who obtains a Residence Order retains his parental responsibility after the order has expired. Step-parents who acquire parental responsibility via a Residence Order lose parental responsibility when the Residence Order ends (Children's Legal Centre, 2005).
- A Specific Issues Order is an order that determines how a specific issue concerning parental responsibility is to be settled. This can be used for decisions about medical treatment (e.g. immunisation, surgery or transplantation, as well as schooling or even deciding in which country a child should live).

*Sections 17–50: Local Authority support for children and families*

These sections include the child protection orders which have been outlined in Chapter 11.

## Adoption and Children Act 2002

This Act changed the law on adoption to bring adoption into line with the Children Act 1989. This Act also altered two aspects of the Children Act 1989 that relate to child health care. These are outlined below. The rest of the Children Act 1989 remains intact.

1. **Domestic violence:** now recognised as a cause of significant harm to children
2. **Parental responsibility:** this changed for any child born after 31 December 2003. Unmarried fathers who register the birth of their child with the mother now have parental responsibility for the child. English law is not retroactive, so the previous regulations apply to children born up until 31 December 2003. Children born under the 1989 regulations can be re-registered if the mother and father both request it. This gives parental responsibility to both parents.
3. **Parental responsibility:** re-registration of the birth using the names of both parents is now possible, enabling the unmarried father to obtain parental responsibility in this way.

## Children Act 2004

This is a significant Act in terms of child protection. It imposes two new duties on agencies, such as NHS trusts, Local Authorities and other public bodies and their employees. The first is the duty to cooperate to safeguard and promote the welfare of children. The second is a duty to safeguard and promote the welfare of children in the normal course of their work. This is why NHS Trusts are offering safeguarding children education to all their staff. This duty also applies where services and resources are contracted out, for example agency staff must have the same level of knowledge as staff employed by the Trust itself. Trust partnership arrangements with universities to educate health professionals imply that students should be provided with child protection education.

## Family Law Reform Act 1969 (Section 8)

This Act allows young people of 16 and 17 years to give valid consent to treatment that is in the child's best interests. It covers surgical, medical or dental treatment and would, by extension, cover nursing care. It includes procedures for the purposes of diagnosis, for example X-ray and anaesthetics. This Act does not take away the parent's power to give consent for a young person of 16 or 17 years of age.

Young people can consent to take part in medical research only where it can be genuinely considered to be part of the treatment of the young person (Dimond, 2005). It excludes taking part in research that will not benefit the child who is involved in the research. It also excludes giving consent for surgery that will not benefit the child. This is particularly relevant in transplant surgery where no one has the right to consent to the removal of an organ from a child which will then be transplanted to another family member – all surgery or procedures must be in the child's best interests.

*Mental Health Act 1983*    This applies to people of all ages, including children. This Act has been under review for some years and new legislation is awaited.

*Data Protection Act 1998*    This defines data in electronic and manual records as confidential and governs what may or may not be disclosed to a third party.

*Human Rights Act 1998*    This enshrines all articles of the European Convention on Human Rights in English law. If someone believes that English law is denying them their human rights, this may be disputed in an English court instead of having to go to the European Court to argue their case.

*Common law*    This is a huge body of case law that has been built up over the centuries. It develops in response to challenges, by individuals, to decisions made in relation to an aspect of statute law or its interpretation.

## CONFIDENTIALITY AND INFORMATION SHARING

Confidentiality and information sharing are two sides of the same coin and cannot be considered without each other. Difficulties arise not in understanding the duty of confidentiality (Dimond, 2005) but in knowing when confidentiality *may* be breached and when confidentiality *must* be breached.

The common law duty of confidentiality has long been part of any professional relationship. In health care it is a requirement of the Nursing and Midwifery Council (NMC) as set out in the NMC's Code of Professional Conduct (NMC, 2004) and is included in the ethical codes of all other healthcare professions. Confidentiality:

- stems from the duty of care owed to patients;
- is implied under a contract of employment or as part of the arrangement between an education provider and practice experience provider for students;
- derives, also, from statute law, in the form of the Data Protection Act 1998 and the Human Rights Act 1998.

In common law, there is a duty to keep confidential information that has been given in confidence, even if there is no legally enforceable contract to that effect. This was only recognised in law in 1988, by the case of *X.* v. *Y. and Another* (2 All ER 648). In this case, a hospital employee, in breach of contract, had leaked the names of two hospital doctors who were being treated for AIDS to a newspaper. The paper published the names and was fined £10 000 following the court's decision that it was not in the public interest to publish information obtained through such a breach of contract.

Detailed government guidance on confidentiality in health care is set out in the *NHS Confidentiality Code of Practice* (Department of Health (DH), 2003). Guidance is not law but government policy spelling out how the law should be interpreted. In April 2006, specific guidance on confidentiality and information sharing relating to children and young people was published following public e-consultation (DfES, 2006a, 2006b). Two flow diagrams from this guidance are given in Appendices 12.1 and 12.2.

## COMMON LAW DUTY OF CONFIDENCE

This exists where there is a special relationship between parties, as in patient and carer. The duty of confidence is not absolute if:

- the information is not confidential in nature – medical records and communications between doctor and patient are confidential; other information may not be (e.g. what time grandparents are coming to visit);
- the person to whom the duty is owed has authorised the disclosure – this could be expressed or implied consent;
- there is an overriding public interest in disclosure (e.g. child abuse, domestic violence, serious crime);
- disclosure is required by a court order or other legal obligation (e.g. police may apply for access to health records under the Police and Criminal Evidence Act 1984 s 9) or a health professional may be ordered (under a subpoena) to appear in court to give evidence in relation to a patient.

Consent to breach confidentiality does not have to be sought if doing so could endanger the child's welfare. Under these circumstances, seeking consent may also prejudice a police investigation or increase the risk of harm to the child. If consent is refused but it is important for the safety of a child to disclose information to a professional, a judgment must be made about whether the disclosure is in proportion to the need to safeguard the child.

Disclosure should be made on a 'need to know' basis. Bear in mind:

- the purpose the disclosure (what will be gained?);
- the nature and amount of information that will be disclosed;
- whether the person receiving the disclosure has a duty to treat the information as confidential;

- whether the benefit of the disclosure is in proportion to the seriousness of the disclosure.

## STATUTE LAW AND CONFIDENTIALITY

The Human Rights Act 1998 article 8 recognises a right to respect for family life (see p. 258, below). The Data Protection Act 1998 regulates the handling of personal data. This information is kept about an individual on a computer or manual filing system. The Act demands that personal data are:

- processed fairly and lawfully;
- obtained only for one or more specified and lawful processes;
- not processed in any way that is not compatible with that or those purposes.

The Data Protection Act 1998 also provides for information sharing, and the conditions for this are very similar to those under the common law duty of confidentiality. They are set out in Schedule 2 (Table 12.1).

These conditions cover most situations where a practitioner shares information to safeguard a child's welfare. A child's physical or mental health or condition is regarded under the Data Protection Act as sensitive personal data, and information sharing is subject to Schedule 3 of the Act. Table 12.2 details some of the conditions of Schedule 3.

The disclosure of confidential information to safeguard the welfare of a child is legal. It is not permissible to disclose confidential information without good reason. An unjustified breach of confidentiality is a civil wrong and may lay you open to being sued for damages.

The following is an example related to confidentiality. A nurse is comparing notes in the staff restaurant with a friend and starts talking about the

**Table 12.1** Schedule 2 Data Protection Act *(Source: HMSO, 1998)*

- The consent of the data subject (the person to whom the data relate) is obtained.
- The disclosure is necessary to comply with a legal obligation.
- It is necessary to protect the vital interests of the data subject.
- It is necessary in the exercise of a statutory function, or other public function exercised in the public interest.
- It is necessary for the purposes of legitimate interests pursued by the person sharing the information, except where it might prejudice the rights, freedoms or legitimate interests of the data subject.

**Table 12.2** Part of Schedule 3 of the Data Protection Act *(Source: HMSO, 1998)*

- It is necessary to protect the vital interests of the data subject or another person and their consent cannot be obtained.
- It is in the substantial public interest and necessary to prevent an unlawful act and obtaining express consent would prejudice those purposes.

teenage boy on the children's ward who is being investigated for HIV. The parent is also in the staff restaurant and overhears this. She knows that there is only one teenage boy on the ward today and is shocked to learn about his possible diagnosis in this way. This is an unjustified disclosure and the Trust may be sued for breach of confidentiality.

Confidential information can be disclosed accidentally in a variety of ways:

- parents overhearing staff conversations and telephone calls (the nurses' station is an especially open invitation to the eavesdropper);
- names of children and consultants written on the bed information board;
- information given to visitors on the assumption that they are the parents – always check first;
- visitors asking questions – a notice stating that health information is confidential and asking visitors not to ask about other children is helpful;
- unauthorised, but 'official looking' people asking for information or looking at notes – if you don't know them, check who they are: are they wearing ID? are they entitled to this information?
- enquiries by phone – how do you know who is actually making the call?

## INFORMED CONSENT AND DECISION-MAKING IN CHILDREN

Any mentally competent adult person has the right in law to consent to anyone touching his or her person. If he or she is touched without consent, they may sue via the civil courts for trespass to the person. This could be battery if they are actually touched and assault if they fear that they will be touched (Dimond, 2005). Serious battery or assault can also be a criminal offence, that can lead to arrest and custodial sentences. The case of re MB (adult medical treatment) [1997] 2 FLR 426 found that a mentally competent adult has the right to refuse treatment for a good reason, a bad reason or no reason at all. An adult may both consent and refuse; the situation is different with children.

Consent and refusal are treated as two different issues in the young. The Family Law Reform Act 1966 (statute law) relates only to consent. In common law, the famous Gillick case also relates to consent, not refusal (Table 12.3).

There is no statute law relating to refusal of treatment, but there is case law. Throughout the 1990s where a child's refusal of treatment has been argued in

**Table 12.3** *Gillick v. West Norfolk and Wisbech Area Health Authority* [1985]

The Gillick case concerned the right of young women below 16 years of age to consent to being given contraceptive advice without their parents knowing. The outcome enables a child of any age to consent to treatment provided that they have 'sufficient understanding and intelligence to understand fully what is proposed'. The principles of the case now cover a much wider area than just contraception.

**Table 12.4** Example cases where children's refusal of treatment has been overridden by the court *(Source: Bijsterveld, 2000)*

---

Re R (1991) – psychiatric medication given to a 15-year-old girl against her will
Re W (1992) – anorexia nervosa, a 15-year-old girl's refusal to move to a specialist hospital
Re E (1993) and Re S (1994) – Jehovah's Witness refusing blood transfusion
Re M (1999) – 15 year-old-girl's refusal of a heart transplant

---

court the child has been ruled to be incompetent to make such an important and life-threatening decision and the refusal has been overruled (Alderson, 2000) (Table 12.4).

Consent is only valid if it is given voluntarily by a mentally competent person, without pressure or fraud. Lack of information on which to make a decision can render the patient's consent invalid and can be seen as a breach of the duty of care on the part of the health professional. To give valid consent for a child, a person must have parental responsibility.

HOW IS CONSENT GIVEN?

Consent is a process. It can only be given when all the necessary details have been explained and a decision reached. This process may take a period of hours or even weeks in relation to surgery. For example, if a girl has repeated throat infections, she knows that she is unwell. She may see the doctor on several or many occasions before being referred to an ear, nose and throat specialist. The referral is made with the permission (consent) of the child and parent, in the knowledge that surgery is a possibility. At the outpatient appointment, discussions take place about possible surgery. The process of consent has begun in earnest against a background of the 'lived' experience of repeated infections and the hope of preventing future episodes of the same illness. The child's name may then go on to a waiting list for surgery before, finally, being called into hospital. Before the child goes to theatre, the parent, and possibly the child as well, give written consent to surgery. There is a whole process of experience and information-giving before a signature is provided. In the case of an emergency, such as a child who has sustained a fracture that needs to be manipulated under an anaesthetic, the timescale is much shorter but the processes of experience and information are generally similar. Consent is much more than a signature. The child needs to be involved all the way through, unless he or she is so young that he or she cannot understand what is going on.

Written consent will be obtained for medical treatment such as a blood transfusion, invasive procedures, for example a lumbar puncture or a barium swallow, and surgery, such as an appendicectomy. However, much of the everyday care given in health services does not require written consent. Verbal or spoken consent is adequate for most of the care interventions made by nurses, therapists and care assistants in caring for the child. The principle of consent is the same. Full information is necessary to enable an informed decision to be made. Sometimes, consent is simply implied: this means there are no words spoken. For example, if you approach a child and ask to take their blood pressure, they may put their arm out for you. This is implied consent. The child has experience of having their blood pressure taken before, understands it and does not need a detailed explanation. If a child has not experienced it before, he or she will need full information about what will happen and in language that they can understand.

Where investigations are concerned, the child, if old enough to comprehend, and the parent need to understand what investigation is being done and why. This may be straightforward if a specimen of urine is to be sent to the laboratory to identify which antibiotic will be effective against an infection. It may become more difficult if the child is 12 years old and the specimen is required for a pregnancy test. This is a routine investigation for girls of this age admitted with abdominal pain, but the child may not understand why such a test is being done and the parents may become offended on the part of the girl and feel that a slur has been cast upon her character. High-level communication skills are required to avoid causing offence, but for consent to be obtained the information must be given.

## YOUNG PEOPLE AGED 16 AND 17 YEARS

### Consent for medical treatment

Section 8 of the Family Law Reform Act 1969 enables 16- and 17-year-olds to consent to medical treatment that is in their best interests. This includes most surgery, investigations and anaesthetics, but excludes piercing or tattooing. It does not take away the right of a parent to give consent for such treatment. Parents may give consent instead of, or in addition to, that of the young person.

### Refusal of medical treatment

Parents can override the refusal of their teenage child. This applies in non-life-threatening cases as well as serious cases. Although, in theory, treatment may be given against the wishes of the young person, few doctors are willing to do this for reasons of ethics rather than law (Bijsterveld, 2000). In less serious cases, for example in plastic surgery where a child does not want to undergo further surgery to neaten a scar, a resolution should be negotiated and the option of future surgery left open. Where the issue is serious or life-threatening, it can be taken to court for resolution. However, 'end of life' decisions to stop active treatment should be discussed openly and negotiated; this is not the same as refusal of treatment.

## YOUNG PEOPLE UNDER 16 YEARS

### Consent to medical treatment

This is known as 'Gillick competence' in law, but often referred to as 'Fraser guidelines' in health care. The professional, usually a doctor, makes the judgment as to whether the child is competent to make the decision or not. Generally, the more serious the decision to be made, the older the child needs to be before being able to give consent.

Defining 'competence to consent' is a difficult and complex task. Although age and intelligence are important factors, so is the child's 'lived' experience of the illness and any previous treatment. Even a small child with a long-term health problem is likely to be able to make some decisions about their treatment and care (Sutcliffe *et al.*, 2004). A child who is involved with decisions made will have a better understanding of what he or she needs to do to help him or her get better. An informed child is much more likely to cooperate with carers and be less anxious than a child who does not know what may be coming next.

### Refusal of medical treatment

Any refusal of life-saving treatment can be overruled by a parent or by the courts. This means that, effectively, a child has no right to refuse life-saving treatment. Where the treatment or investigation is not life-saving and the child is mature enough to reach a decision based on information given, a refusal may be granted. If the investigation is essential, the professional will negotiate a solution that balances patient safety with respect for the individual. This may involve letting the child rest or waiting for a special visitor to arrive if this will not cause harm. These decisions are based on law but also have an important ethical component.

Small children may need to be held still while important investigations, such as venepuncture (taking blood from a vein), are undertaken. The decision to override a child's refusal is taken by the lead professional in the light of the information available at the time. Holding children still and the restraint of children for procedures are ethical as well as practical issues.

## ETHICS

Ethics, sometimes known as morals, are about doing what is right. There are four major ethical principles that are central to health care (Beauchamp and Childress, 2001). These are:

- beneficence (to do good)
- non-maleficence (to do no harm)
- autonomy (making your own decisions)
- justice (treating everyone equally according to their health needs).

'Beneficence' and 'non-maleficence' can be seen as two sides of the same coin, but it is important to try to meet both principles at the same time. This is not always possible. Sometimes, short-term harm may be caused for a long-term benefit. An example of this is causing pain or discomfort to a child with a burn by removing the dressing in order to assess and assist healing. 'Autonomy' is a difficult concept in children, because their ability to make safe decisions is not certain. However, children should be given a choice wherever possible. A small choice about what colour plaster to have is probably better than no choice at all. 'Justice', in health care, is not about punishment but about being fair and treating people equally without prejudice. A very ill child may require more care and time than a less ill child. What makes this just or unjust is whether the patient is treated according to health and social need rather than because the child is particularly endearing or of the same ethnic group as the carer.

Ethical behaviour is usually legal, but sometimes legal actions could be seen as unethical. Both law and ethics need to be taken into account when making decisions about children.

## CHILDREN'S RIGHTS

Children of all ages have the same rights as adults under the Human Rights Act 1998. This Act requires that all English law incorporates the European Convention on Human Rights (1950). The most important components of the Convention in relation to health care can be found in Table 12.5.

Children also have the specific rights set out in the United Nations Convention on the Rights of the Child (UNCRC) (1989). These rights underpin the Royal College of Nursing's (RCN) children's and young person's philosophy of care (RCN, 2003). It is important to note that the UNCRC is not law but has been ratified by the UK – this means that the UK has agreed to abide by it. Children's rights that relate to health care and are not covered by the Human Rights Act 1998 are found in Table 12.6.

## CONCLUSION

The law relating to the health care of children is complex. There is an increasing tension between the rights approach to health care and the welfare (best interests) approach. This may not be obvious in daily care but is noticeable when a dilemma is identified and analysed.

**Table 12.5** European Convention on Human Rights (1950)

| Article | Implications for health care |
|---|---|
| Article 2 – The right to life. This is a fundamental right that cannot be challenged | Killing is unlawful, but treatment may sometimes be withdrawn and a child be allowed to die when further treatment would only cause suffering. This occurs in palliative care when active treatment is withheld but care is provided to keep the child comfortable until death. |
| Article 3 – Prohibition of torture. No one shall be subject to torture or to inhuman or degrading treatment or punishment | Think about your responsibilities to a child in pain, preparing a child for a painful procedure and the dignity of the patient at all times. Consider the way 'holding still' is used during procedures. What is the difference between restraint and holding still? |
| Article 5 – Right to liberty and security of person. Everyone has the right to liberty and security of person | Think about general ward security. Are the children in your care safe? Are there policies in place for the young person who wants to leave the ward, e.g. for a smoke, a walk or to go to the hospital shop? What protects children from being harmed by the people employed to care for them? |
| Article 7 – No punishment without law | Think about discipline of children. Consider some treatments which are more like punishments, e.g. how are children who are drunk or have taken an overdose treated? |
| Article 8 – Right to respect for private and family life, his home and his correspondence | Think of confidentiality as well as the level of privacy available to children and young people in hospital settings. How soundproof are the screens between beds? |
| Article 9 – Freedom of thought, conscience and religion | Children and young people are free to practise their religion if it does not interfere with the rights and freedoms of others. Think about dress codes for children of different religions, e.g. Muslim, Jewish, some Christian sects. |
| Article 10 – Freedom of expression. The exercise of this freedom carries with it duties and responsibilities and may be subject to formalities, conditions, restrictions or penalties prescribed by law | Children and young people are free to express their views, but verbal abuse of others is not acceptable. Children's views of the services should be asked for and acted upon, e.g. the food, the ward environment and facilities and the way their pain was managed. |
| Article 14 – Prohibition of discrimination. No discrimination on any ground such as sex, race, colour, language, religion, political or other opinion, national or social origin, association with a national minority, property, birth or other status | All patients are treated according to their health needs and social care needs. Children's needs are served before their desires, e.g. a family that requires the services of an interpreter probably requires more staff time than a similar family that speak English. What is important is that the child's and family's healthcare needs are met adequately. |

**Table 12.6** Articles of the UNCRC not included in the Human Rights Act 1998

| Article | Implications for health care |
| --- | --- |
| Article 8 – the right to preserve his or her identity | Every child should be treated as an individual, addressed by name, not 'the toddler in bay 2' or 'the boy going to theatre with the broken arm'. |
| Article 9 – a child shall not be separated from his or her parents against their will | Open visiting for parents is the norm. Occasionally, the courts may rule that a parent may not see their child unless accompanied. The mental health team may ask the parents not to visit children and young people who have eating disorders for treatment reasons. This will be identified as part of the young person's care plan. |
| Article 12 – the right to express his or her own views freely, and those views to be given due weight in accordance with the age and maturity of the child | Children should have their views, wishes and feelings heard. Also see the discussion on 'consent'. |
| Article 19 – the right to be protected from all forms of physical or mental violence, injury or abuse, neglect or negligent treatment, maltreatment or exploitation, including sexual abuse, while in the care of parents or any other person who has care of the child | See Chapter 9, for your responsibilities here. Staff need to know the limits of their competence and not take on tasks for which they are not trained. Think about health and safety in every aspect of the care you give and the environment in which it is given. |
| Article 23 – a mentally or physically disabled child should enjoy a full and decent life, in conditions which ensure dignity, promote self-reliance and facilitate the child's active participation in the community | A disabled child is a child first and a patient second. Staff should promote independence as much as possible. |
| Article 24 – the right to enjoy the highest attainable standard of health | This should be the aim of health care. |
| Article 28 – the right to education | During term time, all children of school age are entitled to some education while in hospital. Teachers in hospital often liaise with teachers from the child's own school to enable him/her to keep up with the rest of their class. Public examinations (e.g. GCSE or A levels) may be taken in hospital if children are unable to attend school for health reasons. |
| Article 31 – the right to rest and leisure and play | Play facilities are a vital part of the ward environment (Chapter 8). If you are unsure about whether you should wake a child for observations or not, check with a more senior nurse. Sometimes it is vital that the child is woken; sometimes rest is more important. |
| Articles 32–36 – the right to protection from all forms of exploitation | Research with children is subject to rigorous ethical controls. Photographs of children in hospital may only be used with their permission and that of their parents. Think about visits by celebrities, football teams and the local press. Consent forms are usually required so that there is written evidence that consent for publication has been obtained. |

# REFERENCES

Alderson P (2000) The rise and fall of children's consent to surgery. *Paediatric Nursing* 12(2), 6–8.

Archard D (1993) *Children: Rights and childhood.* London: Routledge.

Beauchamp T and Childress J (2001) *Principles of Biomedical Ethics.* Oxford: Oxford University Press.

Bijsterveld P (2000) Competent to refuse? *Paediatric Nursing* 12(6), 33–35.

Children's Legal Centre (2005) Parental responsibility: frequently asked questions. <http://www.childrenslegalcentre.com> (accessed 5 March 2006).

Department for Education and Skills (DfES) (2006a) *Information sharing: Practitioners' guide.* London: HMSO.

Department for Education and Skills (DfES) (2006b) *Information sharing: Further guidance on legal issues.* London: HMSO.

Department of Health (DH) (2003) *NHS Confidentiality Code of Practice.* London: DH.

Dimond B (2005) *Legal aspects of nursing* (4th edn). Harlow: Pearson Longman.

European Convention on Human Rights (1950) <http://www.echr.coe.int/Library/annexes/CEDH1950ENG.pdf> (accessed 5 March 2006).

Hendrick J (1993) *Child Care Law for Health Professionals.* Oxford: Radcliffe Medical Press.

Nursing and Midwifery Council (NMC) (2004) *The NMC Code of Professional Conduct: Standards for conduct, performance and ethics.* London: NMC.

Royal College of Nursing (RCN) (2003) *Children's and Young Person's Nursing: A philosophy of care.* London: RCN.

Sutcliffe K, Sutcliffe R and Alderson P (2004) Can very young children share in their diabetes care? Ruby's story. *Paediatric Nursing* 16(10), 24–26.

United Nations Convention on the Rights of the Child (1989) <http://www.unhchr.ch/html/menu3/b/k2crc.htm> (accessed 5 March 2006).

Wilkinson R and Caulfield H (2000) *The Human Rights Act: A practical guide for nurses.* London: Whurr.

# CASES

*Donoghue* v. *Stevenson* 1932 AC 562
*E (re) (a minor) (wardship: medical treatment)* [1993] 1FLR 386 FD
*Gillick* v. *West Norfolk and Wisbech AHA* [1985] 3 All ER 402
*M (re) (medical treatment: consent)* [1999] 2 FLR 1097
*M.B. (re) (adult medical treatment)* [1997] 2 FLR 426
*S (re) (a minor) (consent to medical treatment)* [1994] 2 FLR 1065
*W (re) (a minor) (medical treatment)* [1992] 4 All ER 835 CA
*X.* v. *Y. and Another* [1988] 2 All ER 648

## Appendix 12.1. Flowchart of key principles for information sharing

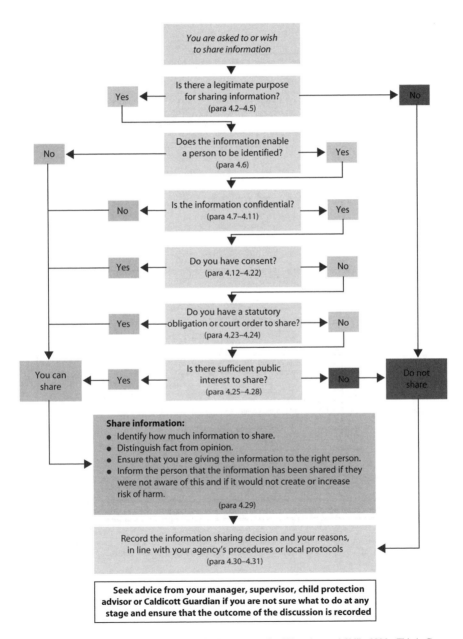

**Flowchart of key principles for information sharing**

Source: *Information sharing: Practitioners' guide.* Department for Education and Skills, 2006a. This is Crown Copyright Material, which is reproduced with the permission of the controller of HMSO and the Queen's Printer for Scotland.

## Appendix 12.2.  Data Protection Act (DPA) 1998 Flowchart

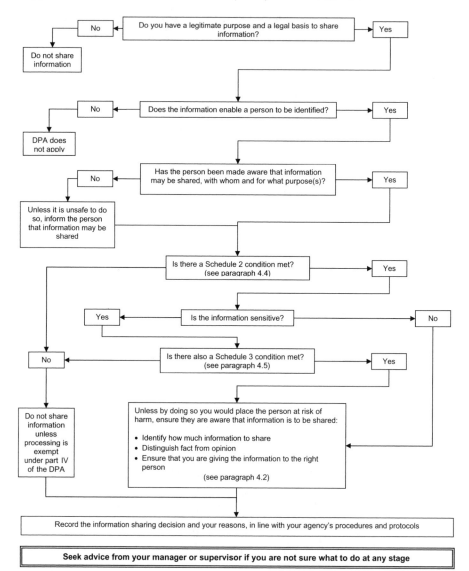

Source: *Information sharing: Further guidance on legal issues.* Department for Education and Skills, 2006b. This is Crown Copyright Material, which is reproduced with the permission of the controller of HMSO and the Queen's Printer for Scotland.

# 13 Future Aspirations

**L. KARSTADT**

## INTRODUCTION

Having now reached the final chapter of this text, you should be well informed about issues relating to caring for children and their families in a healthcare context. You may have been using the book to enable you to underpin your actions within a supporting role, to enhance your studies prior to entry into a nursing or midwifery programme, or as one of many resources used within the earlier stages of professional healthcare education. Whichever of these applies to you, or indeed if you come to this text from another direction, you will need to constantly consider and reconsider where your professional aspirations lie.

This chapter sets out to explore your choices and options for the future. There are a range of occupations in which you may make a significant contribution to the experience of a child and her or his family – sick or well, at home or in hospital. This chapter will discuss both nursing roles and those that complement them. It will also review the facets of professionalism and the way that these relate to children's nurses. Finally, future opportunities for children's nurses will be considered and the possibilities of role changes and modernisation (Department of Health (DH), 2000) will be investigated. Whatever your career ambitions, this chapter should help you to crystallise your ideas and reassure you that the experiences of children are shaped by all those that contribute to their care.

## CHOICES AND OPTIONS

Casey (1988) states that their parents, adequately supported by healthcare professionals, best carry out the care of the child – sick or well. Sick children and their families are in this way supported by a wide spectrum of professionals within hospitals, treatment centres and the community. All these professionals need an adequate knowledge of child development and family dynamics in order to be effective in their job. However, different occupational roles will have different responsibilities and will carry out varying tasks, and therefore preparation is shaped by what families and society expect from the individual

*Caring for Children and Families.* Edited by I. Peate and L. Whiting
© 2006 John Wiley & Sons Ltd

practitioner. For the purpose of this text, roles have been split into two categories: those of professional nurses and others who play a different and complementary role. Both are equally important, although preparation for each occupation is discrete and therefore a person's choice between these two categories is pivotal to their occupational identity in the future.

## NON-NURSING EARLY CHILDHOOD PROFESSIONAL ROLES

The majority of children have spent some time outside the family home by the time they reach their fifth birthday. This may be on a regular or an occasional basis. Positive experiences are guided by well-prepared individuals who are expert in their practice and have the knowledge and skills necessary to guide the development of youngsters in their formative years. The framework for nationally accredited qualifications in early-years education childcare and play work (Qualifications and Curriculum Authority (QCA), 2004) provides a recognition scaffold facilitating progression via the training and opportunities available. Such opportunities are provided in a variety of settings, including community environments such as nurseries and the homes of childminders and hospital environments where children with specific healthcare needs are catered for.

Those who care for small children, whatever their occupation, need core skills. Nursing sick children can be very challenging, and not all individuals are suited to this type of work. Some cope well with the psychological impact of looking after sick children but find the physical challenges difficult. The handling of blood and bodily fluids, or perpetrating painful procedures, does deter some from a career in nursing. Many such individuals still feel, however, that they want to contribute to the care of these children as part of the multidisciplinary team, thus finding an alternative way to support the care and wellbeing of families. In order to operate effectively within the multidisciplinary team, each individual needs to appreciate where they fit in and how their role relates to that of others (Chapter 4). Each team member needs 'the confidence of understanding where the pieces of the jig-saw fit' (Read and Rees, 2000, p. 47). Such non-nurses can, in this way, provide stability and a link with the normal world, and this work is certainly worthy of consideration.

## PROFESSIONAL NURSING OPTIONS

### ADULT NURSING

Those intending to pursue nursing as a career need, at some point, to identify which branch of the profession they wish to join. For some, this will be a straightforward decision, but for others the process will be more difficult with many considerations having to be taken into account. The vast majority of nursing students study the adult branch programme. While being experts in the nursing care of adults, these professionals do still interact with children on several levels. Many adult clients will have small children and so, if these individuals are cared for in the context of their families, interaction with children is unavoidable. This may involve social activity and also the giving of advice where parents wish to involve children in the everyday understanding of health and illness. Similarly, in some clinical areas, although the vast majority of clients are adults, a small number of children may be seen. This is particularly true of places like theatre, accident and emergency units, intensive care units and some outpatient facilities. In an ideal world, children would always be cared for in designated areas and by children's nurses. However, in reality, sometimes children are integrated into a more generic service, where their care is merely overseen by a children's nurse.

Professional nurses working in primary care (that is community care settings) may also interact with children on a regular basis. Practice nurses would normally have an adult nursing background (although children's nurses can undertake this generic position). Additional post-qualification study is generally undertaken to extend the knowledge and capability of the practitioner in order that they may perform this role. In a similar manner, adult nurses can undertake programmes of study leading to a school nurse or health visitor qualification. Both these professionals work primarily with children, and yet, although some will have a children's nurse qualification recorded with the Nursing and Midwifery Council (NMC), it remains a reality that the vast majority have come to this occupation via the adult branch of pre-registration nursing.

If the adult branch is selected, students can expect to undertake a Common Foundation Programme (CFP) which will last for one year followed by a two-year Adult Branch Programme. The initial year enables the student to develop the common knowledge and skills required by all nurses (NMC, 2004a). During this year, half of the student's time will be spent in the university and the balance in practice placement. For students destined to become adult nurses, the vast majority of this time will be spent in practice relating to adult clients. In addition, there will be short alternative experiences which may involve nursing children, patients with mental health problems and clients with a learning disability. Those undertaking the adult branch trajectory can also expect to spend a small amount of time in a maternity placement.

Consequently, during the first year of a nursing programme, all adult branch students can expect to have some interface with children and babies. Once in the branch programme, however, experiences will be exclusively with adults and any interaction with children will be coincidental and unplanned.

CHILDREN'S NURSING

The vast majority of people reading this text will, because of its focus, be attracted to children's nursing. Opportunities to study children's nursing are limited by the number of children found within the health economy, and most universities will restrict their child branch intake to less than 10% of the whole. This means that often there is much competition for places to study children's nursing, which may result in waiting lists or delayed start dates for particular individuals.

Children's nurses are also required to follow the CFP, but can expect to spend a substantial part of their time in placements relating to children. In this context, the short alternative placements will relate to other nursing specialities and will not necessarily include maternity care. This is because the only branch of nursing that is guaranteed reciprocation within the European Union is the adult branch, and to this end adult nursing students are required to reach particular learning outcomes that relate to the maternity experience. The other branches do not require these outcomes. Similarly, under European statute, adult nurses can access a shortened programme of study leading to registration as a midwife (NMC, 2004b). This pathway is not offered to any other branch of nursing. This is unfortunate as most professionals would agree that, given the opportunity, children's nurses would have the potential to benefit from such a shortened course. Given this ruling, any nursing student who thinks that he or she may wish to study midwifery in the future must be advised to undertake the adult branch of nursing.

Children's nursing students will, in their branch programme, extend their clinical experiences with children of varying ages. An individual student can expect to enhance their knowledge and skills with neonates, babies and toddlers, school children and young people. Placements span the health–illness continuum, with different levels of dependency and complexity being experienced within a variety of healthcare settings. By the end of the programme, the student will be proficient in the management and delivery of care of well and sick children. On completion of the pre-registration programme, a menu of post-qualification opportunities in primary, secondary and tertiary care is available. Such nurses can undertake studies that prepare them for the role of health visitor, school nurse, practice nurse or community children's nurse in a primary care context. Alternatively, they can extend other skills that may enable them to advance their careers within the secondary or tertiary care setting.

LEARNING-DISABILITY AND MENTAL HEALTH NURSING

Alongside children's nursing, learning disability and mental health are smaller branches of the pre-registration nursing programme. The learning-disability branch tends to be the smallest and accounts for less than 5% of the total profession. Mental health is larger and accounts for 10–15%. As previously mentioned, all students follow the CFP with a two-year specialised branch programme.

Learning-disability nurses care for clients in all age groups, which, of course, includes children. Within a contemporary society, many children with a learning disability are cared for within the context of their own family. Where this is not possible, children live in small intimate units where family-like care can be provided. Great emphasis is placed upon continuity, and key workers ensure that developmentally each child is enabled to reach her or his potential. It must be emphasised, however, that the vast majority of clients with a learning disability are not children and that those wishing to work exclusively with children should seek specialist advice before making their branch choice.

Similarly, mental health nursing can involve caring for children and young people. Babies are encountered in the mental health context in mother and baby units that deal primarily with women suffering from post-natal depression. Children and young people are, of course, also clients in their own right and provide unique and challenging opportunities for mental health nurses. Additionally, many mental health clients are also parents and this means that such nurses will come into contact with children. Multidisciplinary teams are again pivotal to the management of such clients.

## MIDWIFERY

It has already been stated that the only nurses that have access to shortened pre-registration midwifery programmes are those who have undertaken the adult branch. In addition, students are able to access midwifery by a direct entry route. The number of students following such programmes is governed not only by investment from the NHS but also by the number of maternity patients within the health economy. Each student is required to deliver 40 babies (NMC, 2002a); so the number that any unit can support is finite.

Midwifery education is perceived as very attractive and the direct entry option is oversubscribed in all universities. However, as might be expected, the course is a difficult one in that it prepares participants to practise autonomously. Although the care of the baby is integral to the whole process, applicants must be enabled to view the role of the midwife in its entirety. The challenges of midwifery are numerous and complex and the care of a small baby is an infinitely small part of the whole.

## DIPLOMA OR DEGREE?

Having decided that you want to care for children in a nursing or midwifery professional context, speciality is not your only choice; level of study is also a consideration. The professional qualification equates to registration as a nurse or a midwife and that is what is recorded by the NMC. The NMC maintains a three-part register (Table 13.1).

**Table 13.1** The three parts of the professional register

| Part 1 | Nurse (adult, child, learning disability, mental health) |
| Part 2 | Midwife |
| Part 3 | Community Public Health Nurses |

Registration as a nurse also carries an annotation to indicate whether the individual is an adult, child, learning-disability or mental health nurse.

Alongside the professional qualification, each nurse or midwife will also gain an academic award from the university at which the programme was undertaken. This will be at a minimum diploma in higher education level, but may be an undergraduate BSc or, exceptionally, a postgraduate qualification. Whatever the academic level, the professional qualification is the same and the professional opportunities are similar.

Individuals are encouraged to undertake the programme that best suits their academic ability. Nursing as a profession attracts a wide spectrum of people and this is supported and encouraged both within the profession and in society at large. For those whose formal education ended at 16 years of age and those with no traditional qualifications, the diploma in higher education is the programme of choice. This trajectory introduces university-level education and facilitates a sustained academic development over three years. The complexity of the academic component of this course at completion is comparable with that expected at the end of the second year of a degree programme.

A degree programme, on the other hand, attracts students who have completed A levels or have reached this academic standard by some other means. Over the three years of studying, students reach the same academic level as peers studying degree programmes in other disciplines. In this way, equity of attainment is clearly demonstrated and such nurses are enabled to enter every multiprofessional situation as an equal partner.

Nurses who have undertaken a degree programme are equipped with greater skills of critical analysis and complex decision-making. They also have a greater understanding of the research process. As a consequence of these more developed academic skills, the individual may be well positioned to attain more senior or attractive roles in nurse management, education or research. It should be remembered, however, that many nurses undertaking the diploma initially will go on to achieve a degree after registration. The professional registration is the same whichever academic route is taken and opportunities are usually governed primarily by registration, although additional desirable skills can be facilitated by studying at a higher academic level.

It can therefore be seen that the reader has many choices and options. These relate to whether to pursue a professional nursing and midwifery role or one that is complementary or supportive. Identification of level of study must then be considered. If a professional caring context is chosen, the utmost care must be taken to match personality and career aspirations to career choice. Nursing

**Table 13.2** Some examples of how some registered nurses may work with children in their various roles

| Adult nursing | Children's nursing | Learning Disability nursing | Mental Health nursing | Midwifery |
|---|---|---|---|---|
| Lucy is 25 and has been qualified as a nurse for four years. After completion of the pre-registration programme, she worked in the outpatients department where she cared for patients of all ages including children. After two years, she decided to undertake a BSc programme in Public Health Practice to enable her to work as a health visitor. Lucy's role now is primarily concerned with child health. | On completion of his A levels, Davinda began pre-registration nurse education. After the three-year programme, he elected to work in an acute children's ward in a district general hospital. Nurses on the ward work in partnership with parents to provide care for the sick children therein. Many of the children have respiratory disorders, and the nurses, as part of the multidisciplinary team, prepare families to effectively manage the child's condition at home. | Judith is 28 and entered the learning-disability nursing programme after working in several other jobs. On completion of her studies, she secured a job supporting young families with children with learning disabilities. Her role with these families begins either in the antenatal period, at birth or when the disability is diagnosed. Her role includes health education and practical support for the families in her care. | Philip is 42 and has just qualified as a nurse. Before this, Philip worked as a bank manager but felt that he wanted to do something more fulfilling and give something back to society. His speciality is mental health nursing and his first job as a staff nurse is in an adolescent unit that caters particularly for young people with eating disorders. The work is demanding and many of the young people remain in-patients for months. Their relationship with nurses is pivotal to management. | Fran is 35 and entered the pre-registration midwifery programme aged 28 when her daughter entered full-time education. Fran had enjoyed being pregnant and recognised then that she had many of the personality traits that are required of the good midwife. She enjoys the holistic care of mother and baby and the aspect of her job that prepares the pregnant woman to become a mother. Although Fran likes babies, she would not wish to work exclusively with them. |

offers four options, all of which interface with children to a greater or lesser degree. In addition, midwifery may be chosen, although more than an affinity for small babies is necessary to achieve success. Table 13.2 outlines some possible scenarios with reference to working with children.

## CHARACTERISTICS OF THE PROFESSIONAL NURSE

Once you have decided that the professional nursing or midwifery path is the one that you wish to follow, you must consider how this decision will affect your behaviour in the future. Nursing and midwifery are considered in modern-day society to be professions. This means that the general public and your peer group have certain expectations of you as a professional and that there is a particular body of knowledge and set of competencies that you are expected to acquire prior to registration and to maintain throughout your professional career. The programme of study that you follow, in the first instance, will facilitate/enable the acquisition of the prerequisite knowledge and skills (NMC, 2004a). After registration with the NMC, you will be required to provide periodic evidence that you have kept yourself up to date in relation to your practice proficiency and the knowledge that underpins it.

## THE PROFESSIONAL BODY

The regulating body for nurses and midwives within the United Kingdom (UK) is the NMC. Set up by Parliament, the NMC was established under the Nursing and Midwifery Order (2001) and began to operate in April 2002. Its main function is to protect the public by ensuring that nurses and midwives provide appropriate standards of care to patients and clients. To ensure that this happens, the regulator maintains the professional register. As stated earlier, this consists of three parts: nurses, midwives and community public health nurses (Table 13.1).

The register is a live one with nurses and midwives being required to pay a periodic registration fee every three years. Self-regulation is a tenet of a profession, alongside the autonomous setting of professional standards and having a specific code of professional conduct. Registrants, via the periodic registration fee, fund all of this. The fee in 2005 was under £50 per year and less than that for all other self-regulating healthcare professionals in the UK. In addition to paying the fee, individuals are required to provide evidence that they have kept themselves up to date over the three-year period. A continuing professional development (CPD) portfolio must be maintained by all registrants and can be inspected by the NMC when registration is renewed. Through this process, the NMC exhibits its commitment to lifelong learning.

In addition to maintaining the register, the NMC also considers allegations of misconduct, lack of competence or unfitness to practise owing to ill health. Where such allegations are proven, individuals can be removed permanently, or for an interim period, from the professional register. Removal results in revoking the individual's licence to practise and thus protects the public, as it is illegal to work as a nurse without registration. The NMC also provides advice for nurses and midwives on any professional issue that is challenging them. To this end, the council is not viewed as having a merely punitive function.

Since its inception, the NMC has taken responsibility for the quality and standards within programmes leading to a registerable or recordable nursing and midwifery qualification (NMC, 2004a). Through a network of 'visitors', the NMC ensures that nurses at the point of registration are deemed to be fit for purpose. Visitors also ensure that such programmes have been developed in partnership with the local health economy, embracing both NHS partners and the independent sector, and are viewed by these partners to have the skills required by a registered practitioner.

**Table 13.3** The Code of Professional Conduct *(Source: NMC, 2004)*

As a registered nurse, midwife or specialist community public health nurse, you are personally accountable for your practice. In caring for patients and clients, you must:

- respect the patient or client as an individual;
- obtain consent before you give any treatment or care;
- protect confidential information;
- cooperate with others in the team;
- maintain your professional knowledge and competence;
- be trustworthy;
- act to identify and minimise risk to patients and clients.

These are shared values of all the UK healthcare regulatory bodies.

Standards within programmes of study are only one aspect of the standard setting undertaken by the NMC. In addition, standards relating to conduct performance and ethics are laid down within the NMC's *Code of Professional Conduct* (NMC, 2004c). This code informs registrants of the professional conduct required of them and informs other members of society of the standard of professional conduct they can expect from a registrant (Table 13.3).

The above code of professional conduct underpins everything that an RN does. The values on which the code is based are shared by other professional healthcare workers such as physiotherapists, radiographers and pharmacists and, it could be argued, should be adopted by all who come into contact with children and their families in a caring capacity.

In the context of working with children and families, it is clearly important to interact with the child appropriately. Children's nurses acquire, over the period of their programme of study, a body of knowledge relating to child development and behaviour. They also develop a repertoire of skills to enable them to approach children and their significant carers in a manner that allows them to feel valued and individual. Children's nurses are acknowledged as advocates for both the children in their care and, where appropriate, their families. Within the context of a therapeutic relationship, nurses befriend parents and carers and promote their interests. Holistic care is a central tenet of children's nursing as is the notion of partnership with children and families (Casey, 1995).

Obtaining consent when working with children is just as important as it would be with other client groups. All patients and clients have a right to receive information about their condition (NMC, 2004c). Children must have this information presented to them in a manner conducive to their level of psychological development. The use of storytelling or play should be considered to complement more traditional modes of communication. Children should be involved in all decisions relating to their care, and their consent should always be sought. Obviously, in the case of young children, primarily parents will take important decisions. However, where children can exhibit their competence and the fact that they understand the issues under consideration, they can make autonomous decisions. This is often referred to as 'Gillick competence' or an application of the 'Fraser guidelines' (*Gillick* v. *W Norfolk and Wisbech AHA* [1985] 3 All ER, 402, 423) and has been discussed in Chapter 12 of this book.

The code clearly identifies that all interactions between child, family and nurse are confidential, thus prohibiting private information from being discussed or shared inappropriately. It is not unrealistic to expect this standard of behaviour from anyone whose occupation brings her or him into contact with this vulnerable group. However, sometimes people breach confidentiality inadvertently by discussing families that they are involved with, for example in the dining room, on the bus or in some other public space. This should be guarded against and remains the responsibility of the individual student or practitioner.

The only exception to this confidentiality clause is where the nurse's 'duty of care' overrides their duty to confidentiality. This typically would result where a child or parent discloses evidence of child abuse. In this instance, confidentiality would be broken in order to protect the child (Chapter 11).

The majority of nurses caring for children work in teams. Nursing teams provide stability for children and families both in hospital and in the community. The nursing team is, however, only one part of the group of professionals that will be involved in any one child's care. The code of conduct demands that nurses cooperate with others in the team. This is a pre-requisite if care is to be managed smoothly and everyone is to understand how they fit into the jigsaw (Read and Rees, 2000) of multidisciplinary work. Nurses must be trusted by the children and parents for whom they care and behave in a way that upholds the reputation of the profession. Trust is built up in a number of ways and must be built independently and collectively with the child and their significant adults.

The final item in the list of values concerns the identification and minimisation of risk to patients and clients. This is reliant upon the maintenance of the nurse's unique knowledge base. Using this knowledge, the nurse must work with other members of the multidisciplinary team to promote healthcare environments that are conducive to safe, therapeutic and ethical practice (NMC, 2004c). The first consideration of any nurse must be the interest and safety of the children and families. Where there is suspicion that a colleague may not be fit to practise, an environment is dangerous or standards of care are lacking, the professional nurse has a duty to disclose this information and must be guaranteed protection in relation to the raising of such an issue. As previously discussed, nurses must maintain professional knowledge and competence to remain on the professional register. Such knowledge enables appropriate practice and is dynamic and constantly changing. Updating knowledge underpins contemporary practice and facilitates appropriate decision-making, and so must not be underestimated.

When nurses do not adhere to the code of professional conduct, their professional suitability must be brought into question. In such circumstances, their alleged behaviour would be referred to the NMC and a full investigation carried out. Where appropriate, an individual's name can be removed from the register on a temporary or more permanent basis. The NMC recommends that all practising nurses, midwives and specialist community public health nurses have indemnity insurance. This is in the interests of all parties in the event of claims of professional negligence. Where the employer does not accept vicarious liability on behalf of the employee, it is therefore recommended that the registrant obtain adequate professional indemnity insurance in her or his own right.

## AFTER REGISTRATION

Much has been said about pre-registration education for nurses and midwives. At the point of registration, the individual becomes a practitioner and is expected to practise within the code of professional conduct produced by the NMC (2004c). This is the end of one journey and the beginning of another. Individuals will have chosen the branch in which they wish to practise at the beginning of the programme of study and by the time they register will have a clear professional identity with reference to adult, child, mental health or learning-disability nursing. Further specialisation is, however, almost inevitable. As previously outlined, those who are not primarily children's nurses may position themselves so they have regular contact with children. Other choices will include the focus of practice for an individual and may embrace medical, surgical, palliative care, infection-control, tissue-viability or intensive-care nursing. This list is not exhaustive, and children's nurses can tailor their expertise according to their aspirations.

Practice specialism almost invariably requires specialist education and learning and this usually takes place within a higher education institution (HEI) and is facilitated by nurses who have chosen to develop their careers in an educational context. The NMC records the qualifications that enable nurses and midwives to teach and lays down standards for courses preparing them for this role (NMC, 2002b). Nurse teaching is therefore one recognised career trajectory of the qualified and experienced nurse.

Another trajectory is nursing research. Nurses may be involved in research at a number of levels. They may be part of a team primarily collecting and/or analysing data as directed by others in an already determined fashion. Alternatively, the nurse may work in a team or alone formulating questions, applying for funding, deciding methodology and disseminating findings. All university departments have professors, and nursing departments are no exception. These individuals are established researchers with PhD qualifications who have developed their nursing careers in the context of research.

The vast majority of nurses, however, stay in clinical practice honing and developing their clinical skills throughout their careers. Most work in the hospitals or in the community, as members of a nursing team. For some, the team in which they practise is a multidisciplinary one, to which they will bring a unique nursing perspective. Leadership roles are many and varied and many nurses adopt a management focus as they progress through their careers. This may vary from leading a small team of nurses to directing the nursing service within an acute NHS hospital Trust. Ultimately, some nurses who develop high-level leadership and management skills move outside of a specific nursing context to become hospital general managers or take on board positions that do not require a nursing background.

Nurses, however, do not have to move away from their professional roots in order to be successful. Some nurses maintain a clear nursing identity while developing a largely autonomous and expert role. One such example is the nurse consultant, who has a role that embraces practice, education and research with a focus on client care. Paediatric nurse consultants usually centre their practice on a particular client group. These practitioners are pivotal to the successful management and experiences of particular children and families. Chapter 4 also discusses some of these roles.

## MODERNISATION AND WHAT IT MEANS

*The NHS Plan* (DH, 2000) sets out the vision of a service designed around the needs and aspirations of those who use it. It promises involvement of users and carers and real choice. With the patient or client at the centre of service design and delivery, the hope is to reduce duplication and allow for role re-engineering with the best interests of patients and clients (in our context, children and families) being of primary importance. Obviously, the previous discussion about nurse consultants fits this bill and is seen to be integral to modernisation.

The modernisation effort recognises that, as well as money, changing the way that NHS personnel work and how services are organised is essential to the delivery of real improvement (DH, 2003). Staff are the single biggest resource within the NHS, and the right configuration of staff in optimum numbers allows employers to make the most of this resource and the skills and potential of individual practitioners. *Agenda for Change* (RCN, 2004) sets out to fairly reward nurses and midwives for their efforts, employing the principle of equal pay for work of equal value.

On a local level, this may mean the creation of new hybrid roles with nurses undertaking some tasks or responsibilities previously undertaken by doctors. These include managerial roles, clinical procedures and prescribing. This has become increasingly important in the context of the European Working Time Directive (Council of the EU, 1993), which has seen the hours that doctors are permitted to work reduced. In order to provide a manageable service, other professionals have had to increase the range of their roles to fill the gap. In addition to the advantages of a more flexible service for children and families, individual practitioners extending their responsibilities feel enriched. This improves not only the care received but the way that nurses think about themselves.

Nurses approach the care of children and families in a holistic fashion so that medical tasks are carried out in the context of care and are not as frightening for small children. In addition to medical roles, nurses have also, over recent times, taken back roles that they have not engaged with for decades. Modern matrons take responsibility for cleanliness in acute ward areas and thus make an enhanced contribution to the wider patient experience, for example the reduction of infection. All targets for modern matrons have been exceeded, and these individuals are becoming significant players in local Trusts. Community matrons are also now being considered. Similar to their hospital counterparts, these individuals will take responsibility for chronic disease and caseload management. They will usually work with the elderly or chronically sick, although a small number of very specialist roles may be available to children's nurses.

In reality, modernisation in the context of those working in the NHS with children has meant more roles that support children and families both within acute hospital Trusts and in the community. Such roles have been made available at registrant level and in some parts of the country at assistant practitioner level. As with nurse consultant roles, most new roles are engineered around particular client groups, like those with cystic fibrosis or epilepsy. Delivery of an appropriate service with the child and family at the centre is pivotal to modernisation and the notion that practice and services can be still further improved.

## IN THE FUTURE

As previously mentioned, children's nurses historically, in the UK, have had their own part of the professional register. With the setting up of the new register, referred to earlier in this chapter, this is no longer the case. Children's nurses now have an annotation beside their name to indicate that they have been specially prepared to work with this client group. This new arrangement may offer some innovative opportunities for educational institutions to offer original programmes that prepare practitioners to relate to more than one client group. For example, universities may organise their courses so that they prepare nurses to work with clients of any age, and consequently have their name annotated with both adult and children's nursing symbols on the professional register.

Similarly, some institutions may seek to create new roles, such as family nurses, for whom the question of registration may prove a challenge that will have to be addressed alongside the programme development. Again, opportunities may be presented in a professional or complementary context. Generic workers have been mooted for a number of years. Such individuals could cross professional boundaries so that they undertake roles traditionally undertaken by nurses, therapists, social workers and others. Their creation would be needs led. These individuals could be at advanced practitioner, practitioner or assistant practitioner level. In the spirit of modernisation (DH, 2000), the experience and well-being of the client would be seen as the policy driver.

## CONCLUSION

In conclusion, those wishing to work with children and families have a number of choices and options, in a professional or non-professional context, within the health service and outside it. Having read this chapter and internalised some of the expectations of a professional, you should now be in a position to make a decision. Those that choose to embark on a professional trajectory within a professional NHS can expect to be challenged. The rewards, however, are immense and inclusion in the global family of nursing has for many of us been an enriching and salutary experience.

## REFERENCES

Casey A (1988) A partnership with child and family. *Senior Nurse* 8(4), 8–9.
Casey A (1995) Partnership nursing: Influences on involvement of informal carers. *Journal of Advanced Nursing* 22, 1058–1062.
Council of the European Union (1993) Council Directive No. 93/104/EC.
Department of Health (DH) (2000) *The NHS Plan: A plan for investment, a plan for reform.* London: TSO.
Department of Health (DH) (2003) *The NHS Plan: A progress report. Modernisation Board Annual Report 2003.* London: TSO.
Nursing and Midwifery Council (NMC) (2002a) *Requirements for Pre-registration Midwifery Programmes.* London: NMC.
Nursing and Midwifery Council (NMC) (2002b) *Standards for the Preparation of Teachers of Nursing and Midwifery.* London: NMC.
Nursing and Midwifery Council (NMC) (2004a) *Standards of Proficiency for Pre-registration Nurse Education.* London: NMC.
Nursing and Midwifery Council (NMC) (2004b) *Standards of Proficiency for Pre-registration Midwifery Education.* London: NMC.
Nursing and Midwifery Council (NMC) (2004c) *Code of Professional Conduct.* London: NMC.
Nursing and Midwifery Order (2001) *(SI 2002/253).* Norwich: TSO.
Qualifications and Curriculum Authority (2004) *The Statutory Regulation of External Qualifications in England Wales and Northern Ireland.* London: QCA.

Read M and Rees M (2000) Working in teams in early years setting. In: R Drury, L Miller and R Campbell (eds) *Looking at Early Years Education and Care.* London: David Fulton.

Royal College of Nursing (RCN) (2004) *Agenda for Change: Getting prepared.* London: RCN.

# Glossary of Terms and Abbreviations

*advocate*  an individual who acts as mediator or speaks for another person.

*anaemia*  the reduction of red blood cells or the reduction of the oxygen carrying pigment haemoglobin.

*ANTT*  aseptic non-touch technique.

*apnoea*  temporary cessation of breathing, a respiratory pause of more than 20 seconds.

*ASH*  Action on Smoking and Health.

*assessment data*  findings, objective or subjective, that can be used to make judgments/inferences regarding the health and social circumstance of an individual.

*assessment tools*  a variety of frameworks available to allow the assessment of individual needs.

*astigmatism*  a defect of vision. Images of objects become distorted as a result of unequal curvatures in the cornea or lens.

*bronchiolitis*  inflammation of the bronchioles.

*CAPT*  Child Accident Prevention Trust.

*CAT scan*  computer axial tomography scan.

*CFP*  Common Foundation Programme.

*child abuse*  a broad term used to include neglect, physical injury, sexual or/and emotional abuse of a child usually, but not exclusively, by adults.

*CMO*  Chief Medical Officer.

*CNO*  Chief Nursing Officer.

*community children's nurse*  a children's nurse who has been specifically educated and has the skill, knowledge and attitudes to provide care for the child and family in a community environment (e.g. home, school).

*conductive hearing loss*  hearing loss from interference of transmission of sound to the middle ear.

*confidentiality*  the duty to keep any information private, or limit its release to specified individuals.

*cooperative play*  children who play in a group with their peers in one organised activity that has rules and goals.

*coryza*  acute inflammation of the nasal mucous membrane accompanied by a profuse nasal discharge.

*CNST*  Clinical Negligence Scheme for Trusts.

*Caring for Children and Families*. Edited by I. Peate and L. Whiting
© 2006 John Wiley & Sons Ltd

*CPD*   continuing professional development.

*culture*   dynamic and integrated structures of knowledge, beliefs, behaviours, ideas, attitudes, values, habits, customs, language, symbols, rituals, ceremonies, and practices that are unique to a particular group of people.

*cyanosis*   a bluish discoloration of the skin and mucous membranes, e.g. lips.

*development*   progressive increase in the ability to function.

*DfES*   Department for Education and Skills.

*DH*   Department of Health.

*diarrhoea*   an increased frequency or a decreased consistency of stools.

*diastole*   period between two contractions of the heart. Occurs when the muscle of the heart relaxes allowing the chambers of the heart to fill with blood.

*DTI*   Department of Trade and Industry.

*dyspnoea*   difficulty in breathing.

*ECG*   electrocardiogram.

*electrolyte*   solutions that produce ions, i.e. sodium ($Na^+$).

*empowerment*   providing or giving control and/or authority to another.

*evaluation*   reassessment in order to determine the effects of interventions (i.e. nursing interventions).

*EPO*   Emergency Protection Order.

*family-centred approach to care*   the needs of all the family are considered in health or illness.

*fat soluble vitamins*   vitamins A, D, E and K.

*febrile convulsion*   a seizure associated with a rapid increase in temperature in younger children (six months–five years).

*FGM*   female genital mutilation.

*FSID*   Foundation for Sudden Infant Death.

*growth*   progressive increase in physical size.

*GP*   general practitioner.

*haemoglobin*   oxygen carrying pigment containing iron, found in red blood cells.

*HCA*   healthcare assistant.

*HASS*   Home Accident Surveillance System.

*HDA*   Health Development Agency.

*HEI*   higher education institution.

*holistic*   attending to the needs of the whole person, considering their mental, social and physical needs.

*HO*   house officer.

*HSE*   Health and Safety Executive.

*hypoxia*   reduction in the availability of oxygen to the tissues.

*ICO*   Interim Care Order.

*ICU*   intensive care unit.

*informed consent*   providing those concerned (i.e. the child and her/his family) with the necessary competence to consent to a procedure that they can understand. The child/parent must fully understand the proposed treatment as well as the possible risks and benefits.

*myopia*   ability to see objects clearly at close range but not from a distance – short sightedness.

*MRI*   magnetic resonance imaging.

*MRSA*   methicillin-resistant *Staphylococcus aureus*.

*NAO*   National Audit Office.

*NICE*   National Institute for Health and Clinical Excellence.

*NMAS*   Nursing and Midwifery Admissions Service.

*NMC*   Nursing and Midwifery Council.

*non-accidental injury*   a non-accidental traumatic incident that produces physical and/or psychological harm.

*PALS*   Patient Advice and Liaison Services.

*partnership*   sharing and taking part with another or others.

*parallel play*   children play next to, but not necessarily with, one another; they may engage in separate activities and in general they do not share rules, goals or purpose.

*PAU*   paediatric assessment unit.

*PCT*   Primary Care Trust.

*PICU*   paediatric intensive care unit.

*play therapy*   a technique used by trained therapists to interpret through play the behaviours of an emotionally disturbed child.

*PPO*   Police Protection Orders.

*RCN*   Royal College of Nursing.

*SCBU*   special care baby unit.

*SHA*   Strategic Health Authorities.

*SHO*   senior house officer.

*solitary play*   children who do not seek out the company of others to play.

*SpHA*   Special Health Authorities.

*SpR*   specialist registrar.

*SR*   senior registrar.

*systole*   the period of contraction of the heart – in particular the ventricles.

*therapeutic play*   usually purposeful and structured, led by an adult with the intention of monitoring the holistic well being of the child.

*trauma*   physical wound or injury, or emotionally painful or harmful event.

*UCAS*   Universities & Colleges Admissions Service.

*UKCC*   United Kingdom Central Council for Nursing, Midwifery and Health Visiting.

*water-soluble vitamins*   B complex and C vitamins.

# Index

ABC 130, 134
abduction 226
absorption 109, 111, 112, 115, 122
abuse 224–39, 259, 279
  child protection 222–3, 224–39
  confidentiality 251, 261
  emotional 226, 227, 229–30
  neglect 226, 227, 231
  NMC 272
  physical 226, 227–9
  sexual 225–7, 231–3, 234–5, 259
*Access to Nursing* 1
accident and emergency departments
  16, 55, 127, 207–8
  breathing 140
  nursing career options 265
  play 167
  teams and teamwork 69
accidents 4, 11, 76, 192, 203–18
  child protection 227–8
  government policy 215–16
  medication 173–4
  play 160
  rates 204
accountability 175, 176
Action for Sick Children (ASC) 13
Activities of Living Model 132
acute care 54, 55, 56, 59, 114
acyanotic heart defects 96–7, 121
adenoids 118, 139
adjourning stage of teams 64
adolescence 7, 43, 61, 255, 269
  accident prevention 205, 206, 207–8
  child protection 235
  consent 255
  drawing 35
  health promotion 74, 82, 83–4

legal concerns 244
play 157, 166–7
adoption 8, 221, 248
Adoption and Children Act (2002)
  249
Adult Branch Programme 265
adult nursing 264–5, 273
  career options 264–9, 273
advanced practitioners 276
adverse events 171–2, 173, 177
advocacy 44, 174, 279
age 7, 11, 13, 15, 19, 144, 255–6
  accidents 4, 204–10, 214, 216–18
  administration of medication 173, 174,
    179
  assessment 126, 129, 152
  blood pressure 144, 145–6
  breathing 133, 134, 140, 142
  child protection 230, 232–5, 237–8
  circulatory system 95
  communication 26, 31, 32, 33, 44
  consent 253–4, 255–6
  digestive system 110
  drawing 34, 35–41
  febrile convulsions 108–9
  health promotion 74, 75, 79–81, 84
  immune system 105
  legal concerns 244, 246, 248–50, 253–6,
    259
  maternal 209, 214
  moving and handling 193
  play and development 156–61, 164–6
  respiratory system 101, 103, 104
  temperature 106, 147, 149, 150
  toddlers 29–33, 35
  UNCRC 259
*Agenda for Change* 274

*Caring for Children and Families.* Edited by I. Peate and L. Whiting
© 2006 John Wiley & Sons Ltd